CANDIDA ALBICANS

By the same author:
Allergies
Arthritis
Eczema and Psoriasis
Irritable Bowel Syndrome
Menopause
Stress
Weight Control

CANDIDA ALBICANS

HOW YOUR DIET CAN HELP

Stephen Terrass

Thorsons

An Imprint of HarperCollins*Publishers*

Thorsons
An Imprint of HarperCollins*Publishers*
77–85 Fulham Palace Road,
Hammersmith, London W6 8JB
1160 Battery Street,
San Francisco, California 94111–1213

Published by Thorsons 1996

10 9 8 7 6 5 4 3 2 1

A catalogue record for this book
is available from the British Library

ISBN 0 7225 3150 8

Printed in Great Britain by
Caledonian International Book Manufacturing Ltd, Glasgow

To Nicola, whose love, understanding, patience, encouragement and valuable input have helped me immeasurably in the writing of this book.

CONTENTS

ACKNOWLEDGEMENTS

The author wishes to thank the following for their valuable support and assistance in this project: Richard Passwater Ph.D. for his inspiration and reviewing of the manuscript; editors Jo Kyle and Wanda Whiteley, and copy-editor Barbara Vesey; Eileen Campbell and Jane Graham-Maw for their help and commitment to this series; Michele Turney, Geoff Duffield and Megan Slyfield for their hard work and dedication; William Crook M.D. for his generosity; special thanks to Rand Skolnick, John Steenson, Cheryl Thallon, Fay Higginbotham and Leyanne Scharff for their valuable support; and all my friends from health food stores and colleagues in the natural medicine field. Most of all, fondest thanks to Nicola Squire and Shirley Terrass for their love and encouragement.

Over the past several years there has been an ever-increasing interest in health matters. It is not really that this is such a new phenomenon; what is new, though, is the focus on 'doing it yourself' rather than merely relying on someone else to keep you in one piece, so to speak. It would be naïve to suggest that this trend involves the majority of people in Western society today, but the movement toward self-reliance is certainly encouraging – especially to those involved in the field of natural medicine and health care.

Holistic health refers to treating the whole person, rather than just his or her symptoms, and it provides sufferers with an incredible springboard to taking responsibility for their own physical well-being. For practitioners of natural and holistic health it offers a wonderful opportunity to help people help themselves. This is a major step toward achieving not just a healthy body but overall health and happiness – surely a goal to which we all aspire.

It is not that society does not need symptomatic treatments, drug therapies or orthodox medicine; there are times when these are vital, even life-saving. However, the only guaranteed cure for any disease or disorder is *prevention*, and prevention is only entirely in your own hands.

Many adopt a healthier lifestyle because they assume

that it is bound to pay dividends eventually, but they are not exactly sure what to expect. Others try to live a bit more healthily than the average person, all the while wondering whether their efforts are just a way of making them feel good about themselves. Fortunately, there is a huge amount of medical and scientific research which proves beyond a shadow of a doubt that many different preventative health approaches do actually work in a measurable way. Research journals are littered with study after study which validate this point. These proven approaches, whether they are for preventing heart disease, cancer, arthritis, osteoporosis, etc. tend to focus on dietary changes, lifestyle factors, nutritional supplementation, herbal medicine and stress-reduction techniques – and these methods have been found to be valuable in the treatment of countless health disorders.

Naturally the greatest focus within the medical and scientific community is going to be on the most well-known and highly publicized health problems, but there are many others which are more common than many people realize or would ever suspect. As a matter of fact, there are examples of health disorders which are proven to be relatively common that are frequently ignored by orthodox medicine. There is, perhaps, no better example of this than the common syndrome candidiasis, caused by the yeast *Candida albicans*. It is thanks to the ground-breaking revelations of C. Orian Truss M.D., followed soon after by the work of William Crook M.D., that more and more practitioners, scientists and members of the general public are becoming familiar with the nature and extent of this disorder. The information in this book is designed to help you to gain control over this all-too-common contributor to ill health.

Over the last few years I have had the pleasure of review-ing the manuscripts of the eight books written to date by Stephen Terrass. One might assume that as a scientific researcher and author, the last thing I would like to do is read yet another health book! However, as is the case with all his books, *Candida Albicans* is not just another health book. Stephen has achieved the very delicate balance needed to make what are often intricate and confusing health issues accessible to the reader. They are scientifically based without being too technical. They are well organised and enjoyable to read without deviating from the subject at hand.

In *Candida Albicans* Stephen tackles one of the most intriguing of health disorders, chronic candidiasis, some-times known as the 'yeast syndrome'. The awareness of Candida is not new; it is the yeast organism responsible for the common thrush infection. However, this yeast is found in the intestines of every person, and the possibility of it causing a syndrome with an almost unlimited scope is a concept which would arouse the curiosity of any scientist.

As it happens, the 'yeast syndrome' is no longer just a concept, in some people it is a reality. Unfortunately, the orthodox medical community has been very slow to accept what the medical literature has been telling us for some time now; that given the opportunity, *Candida albicans* can spread beyond its normal confines and invade most any part of your body, directly or indirectly, causing a vast array of symptoms and altering any body system. This lack of acceptance is especially distressing when you consider the fact that the use of prescribed antibiotics, steroids, birth control pills, etc. represent the most likely causes of Candida getting out of control in the first place.

Fortunately, in this book Stephen Terrass unravels the confusing yet fascinating subject of candidiasis; from its causes, symptoms and possible effects on the body, to a practical and natural treatment protocol based on the latest scientific research. Whether you are debilitated by the effects of the yeast syndrome throughout your body, or are only affected by the occasional thrush infection, this book is a must!

Richard A. Passwater Ph.D.
Berlin, Maryland, USA
March 1996

Do you suffer with chronic digestive problems such as bloating, diarrhoea and/or constipation, nausea, gas or indigestion? Are you stricken with regular headaches, light-headedness or depression? Do you seem to be tired all the time no matter how much sleep you get? Have you been experiencing an abnormally severe craving for cakes, candies and anything sweet? Are you unusually sensitive to foods, perfumes or pollution? Have you managed to catch seemingly every virus which comes within breathing distance? Do you have little or no tolerance for stress? Do you regularly have dark circles under your eyes, and does your skin lack that healthy glow? Are you prone to severe premenstrual or menstrual difficulties? Have you experienced repeated vaginal irritation, prostatitis or thrush infections? Have you undergone repeated or long-term use of antibiotics, birth control pills or corticosteroids?

If the answer to even a few of these questions is 'yes', then there may be a great deal to be gained from this book. If many of the questions apply to you then you should study the information in the chapters that follow very carefully indeed, as there is a good chance that your problems are related to the yeast *Candida albicans*.

In Western society today, threats such as cancer, AIDS and heart disease have understandably been at the forefront of people's concerns, in part due to the heavy media attention which has been centred on them, campaigns by health groups and charities, and so on. The fear which they engender also accounts for their high profile. What are deemed as less serious health concerns, such as arthritis or premenstrual tension, get a lot of attention as well, probably due to their prevalence among 'ordinary' people with 'average' lifestyles. *Candida albicans* is far from a household term, but more and more people are becoming familiar with it due to the growing publicity about its potentially damaging effects.

The existence of *Candida albicans* has been documented in research for several decades. Also well documented is the fact that *Candida albicans* is perfectly capable of causing health problems should it happen to get out of control. For the most part, the entire focus of orthodox medicine on this potentially harmful yeast has been with respect to the localized yeast infection known as thrush. Unfortunately, there is a great deal of evidence which shows that the scope of candida-related problems spans far wider than a temporary case of thrush. As a matter of fact, literally every part of the body can be adversely affected by *Candida albicans*.

The list of symptoms which can be associated with candidiasis is immense, as is the list of other health disorders which can either be caused or influenced by it. For so many people, the syndrome known as candidiasis has become the most distressing challenge to their physical and emotional health that they have ever experienced, not least because they are likely to have run into countless 'brick walls' before they could even find someone to identify the cause of their ill health in the first place. Of course, this means that there are many, many others out there whose problems are being caused by this yeast yet who may never be properly diagnosed.

In spite of this, there is good news. The awareness of candidiasis and the potential of this yeast to damage health is becoming increasingly accepted by the medical community. Actually, the natural medicine community has taken the subject very seriously ever since candida was shown to have more than just a localized influence, and this community still offers the greatest access to beneficial therapies and information. The greater acceptance of the magnitude of candidiasis is encouraging even more research, which is uncovering many new developments in the successful treatment of this condition.

Whenever you suffer with a health disorder the first priority is proper diagnosis. With respect to treatment, it is not only important to be aware of the symptoms, but vital also to understand the likely causes of the condition. Understanding and then addressing the cause or causes yields the best possible chance of successful treatment, not to mention prevention in the future. All these factors represent the focus of this book. First we will look at the background and definition of *Candida albicans* and the syndrome of candidiasis. Within this discussion will be an explanation of the digestive environment and the manner in which candida emerges from its normal habitat in the intestines to wreak havoc on other parts of the body. The symptoms of candidiasis in its many forms will also be discussed. We will also focus on learning about the potential causes of the condition and of other health disorders which are very closely linked to candidiasis. Finally you will learn how to use dietary management and nutritional and herbal supplementation as a safe, effective and scientifically proven approach to treating candida-related health problems.

Do you suspect you suffer with candidiasis? Have you

been diagnosed with candidiasis but have been thus far unsuccessful in winning the battle against it? Do you feel unwell almost all the time and don't know why? Are you sick and tired of being sick and tired? This book may help you to discover what is wrong. If candidiasis turns out to be your problem, then the information that follows will uncover methods you can use to defeat it and reclaim full health in the process.

Note: The dietary and health recommendations in this book are meant only as guidelines. Neither the author nor the publishers can assume responsibility if any of the dietary or lifestyle recommendations in this book do not have the desired effect. Please consult a qualified health practitioner before embarking on any new diet or health regime.

PART 1

Candidiasis and Its Development

CHAPTER 1

What Is *Candida Albicans*?

Undoubtedly you are familiar with the concept of disorders caused by unwanted 'germs' due to personal experience of the common cold, influenza and the like. The publicity about HIV and AIDS has ingrained in us the fact that some of these organisms are particularly lethal. For the most part, the emphasis has been on viruses and harmful bacteria. However, there are many other types of living organisms which can do untold damage to your body. Certain parasitic organisms can cause illnesses ranging from relatively mild disorders (such as travellers' diarrhoea) to quite severe ones (such as malaria). The organism *Candida albicans* is yet another which represents a very real threat to health.

DEFINITION

Candida albicans is a type of yeast which belongs to the family of organisms known as fungi. There are countless species of this family in nature and they can be found most anywhere. Because they are living organisms all they need is a minimally suitable environment in which to take up residence.

Members of the fungi family are unusual in their ability to survive in environments which are unsuitable for so many others. An example that you will be most familiar with is mushrooms, which enjoy a dark, moist habitat and can live off most anything. Their survival owes a great deal to the fact they do not need to take up roots to feed and they can thrive on countless types of organic matter. Fungi are not only found in your garden, however. They also grow within your body, and are doing so this very instant, for instance in the form of *Candida albicans*. Of course, candida is not a mushroom; it is originally comprised of a tiny single yeast cell. As with all yeast cells or spores, they multiply to form new cells which will multiply in turn – the possible result being an exponential growth of the single yeast cell into a yeast colony. This is, of course, another great asset to survival of their species.

Actually, you are full of several pounds of different organisms which have taken up residence in or on your body without your permission. While this thought may make your skin crawl, it should be comforting to know that many of these organisms have formed a *mutually beneficial* relationship with human beings. This symbiotic partnership obliges you to provide the 'friendly' organisms with a home and a steady meal, so to speak. They in turn assist you in some metabolic processes and provide a security patrol against other tiny visitors which vandalize the very environment which gives them shelter. (In this book we will use the term *pathogenic* to refer to potentially disease-causing organisms.) While fungi actually serve a beneficial purpose in nature, such as aiding in the decomposition of dead organic matter, when yeast cells of *Candida albicans* proliferate in your body, they serve no known helpful function. As a matter of fact, if allowed to run rampant they can do untold damage to essentially any part of your body. The relationship between you and these organisms will be discussed in much more detail throughout this book, as this issue not only helps explain how candida adversely affects the body, but also how it can be controlled.

The primary site of the proliferation of micro-organisms in your body is the intestinal tract. This is also the case for *Candida albicans*, although if circumstances allow, candida will happily multiply and its new numbers will migrate to other areas which are hospitable to its survival. The reasons for its spread and the implications of any unchecked multiplication will be discussed in Chapters 4 and 5.

It is precisely at this point of unchecked multiplication and migration that candida yeast cells account for the real issue that this book intends to address – *candidiasis*. Candidiasis, sometimes referred to as 'the yeast syndrome', is the condition whereby *Candida albicans* vastly increases in numbers, spreads beyond its normal habitat in the lower intestine and causes a vast array of symptoms, often either leading to or exacerbating existing health disorders.

Systemic Candidiasis

Candidiasis varies considerably in its severity from one person to the next. In some people, the candida will overgrow within limits and cause a local manifestation, such as in the case of vaginal thrush. In others, the more severe situation arises where the candida travels far beyond the abdominal region and begins to infiltrate the bloodstream in large numbers. This allows candida to affect adversely literally every part of the body – a condition known as *systemic candidiasis*. Although not inevitable, systemic candidiasis is common in those who suffer repeatedly with less severe bouts of candidiasis. Some people can develop a systemic yeast infection even if they have not suffered with yeast problems in the past.

Fungal Form of Candida

Candida's transition from a local to a systemic infection is one of its most fascinating, albeit disturbing, aspects. In its normal state, candida is a simple yeast cell (blastospore). Unfortunately, it has the unique ability to convert into what is known as a *mycelial fungal form*, which has a considerably greater scope for destruction than the simple yeast form. This insidious process involves the production of a 'root' sprouting from the cell, called a *hypha*.

When the newly formed hypha sprouts branches it becomes a *mycelia*. The additional destructive capabilities afforded to candida are due to the hypha (root) and mycelia (its branches).

When a person is in good health, normally the mucus lining of the intestinal wall provides a reasonable barrier to inhibit the passage of unwanted substances into the bloodstream. Unless there are significant adverse changes to the integrity of the intestinal barrier (as often occurs in chronic candida overgrowth), the simple yeast form of candida finds it difficult to permeate the intestines. The fungal transition, however, supplies the answer to this dilemma – to candida's ultimate benefit (and the sufferer's detriment). The root structure allows the candida to penetrate this mucosal defence that lines the intestinal tract (and/or the vaginal canal in women), thereby gaining easier access to your entire system. Nutritional methods of deterring the fungal transition will be discussed in Chapter 9.

No matter whether candidiasis is systemic or more isolated, early diagnosis is very important to stemming the tide of damage and suffering. After all, *Candida albicans* is essentially a parasite, with an inborn drive to feed, multiply and spread. Fortunately, successful control and treatment can be achieved, but only if you know for sure what you are dealing with.

DIAGNOSIS

It is unfortunate that the awareness of the damaging effects of *Candida albicans* is still in its relative infancy among most of the orthodox medical community. It is not known how many of us suffer with the implications of unchecked *Candida albicans* overgrowth and spread, but it *is* known how many of us have *Candida albicans* in our body – *everyone*. All adults and all but a small percentage of infants have *Candida albicans* in their bodies; yet not all of us suffer with candidiasis, systemic or otherwise. Ironically, it is probably the ubiquitous nature of candida that is the very reason why so little is known by orthodox doctors as to its range of effects.

Laboratory Tests for Candida

There are a couple of diagnostic procedures which will verify the presence of *Candida albicans* in the body, such as stool cultures and testing for antibodies to candida. As candida mainly inhabits the intestines, it will typically be present in stool samples, and thus is unlikely to 'raise any sirens' to alert the doctor that something is amiss. When an invader gets into the bloodstream the body's defence force, the immune system, will often produce antibodies which trigger a chain reaction that destroys the foreign substance. As it turns out, almost everyone has antibodies to *Candida albicans*, showing that it has one way or another moved beyond its normal environment in the intestines. A strong immune system can destroy the infiltrating candida before it creates havoc, but as you will soon see, it is often a weakened immunity which allows it to harm the body so thoroughly. In any event, as with stool cultures, the mere presence of candida antibodies may not seem all that alarming to a technician who comes across them in a blood test.

Hence, the two most 'scientific' methods of verifying the presence of candida in the body may seem a bit redundant. After all, it would seem pointless to diagnose the *presence* of candida when we all have it, and it is not the mere existence of candida which is harmful anyway. The tests are not useless, however, as an abnormally large concentration of candida in the stool or a high concentration of candida antibodies may provide a useful clue to diagnosis. However, what is most important is to diagnose whether candida is responsible for the series of symptoms a person may be suffering with, and the lab tests will not be able to confirm this on their own.

Diagnostic Questionnaires

A well-designed questionnaire, on the other hand, can be very helpful in assessing the likelihood that your symptoms are caused by candidiasis. The many different candidiasis questionnaires that have been produced over the years may not be perfect, but they are probably a more suitable gauge of candida-related health problems than lab diagnosis alone. Optimally both a questionnaire and laboratory procedures will be used together to provide a guide to diagnosis. In Chapter 6 there is an example of a candidiasis questionnaire which you can use in the first instance.

As the primary site of activity of *Candida albicans* is the intestines, in order to grasp fully how candida gets out of control and can cause its vast and very disturbing range of symptoms, the next chapter focuses on the structure and function of the digestive tract, providing information that will be referred to repeatedly throughout the rest of this book.

CHAPTER 2

The Digestive System

The health of the digestive system, or lack thereof, significantly affects every cell in the body and can be a major determining factor in a great many health disorders. Much of the activity of micro-organisms takes place in the digestive system – reason enough to concentrate on maintaining its health. Even in the case of health disorders where the digestive tract is not so directly involved, it is still important to ensure that this system is working properly.

THE DIGESTIVE PROCESS

The digestive process involves the breakdown of the food you eat into a form which can be used to nourish your body's trillions of cells. The basic premise of digestion is nothing new to us, but the more intricate processes are very complex. As is the case in life in general, the more complicated a process of human biochemistry is, the easier it is for things to go wrong. Digestion involves more than turning solid food into a less solid form, and should the digestive process not be completed the food you eat will be useless in providing what your cells require in order to function.

Nutrients from Food

The foods you eat are made up of various components which can be used by the body for nourishment. These components, known as *nutrients*, are used by the body for

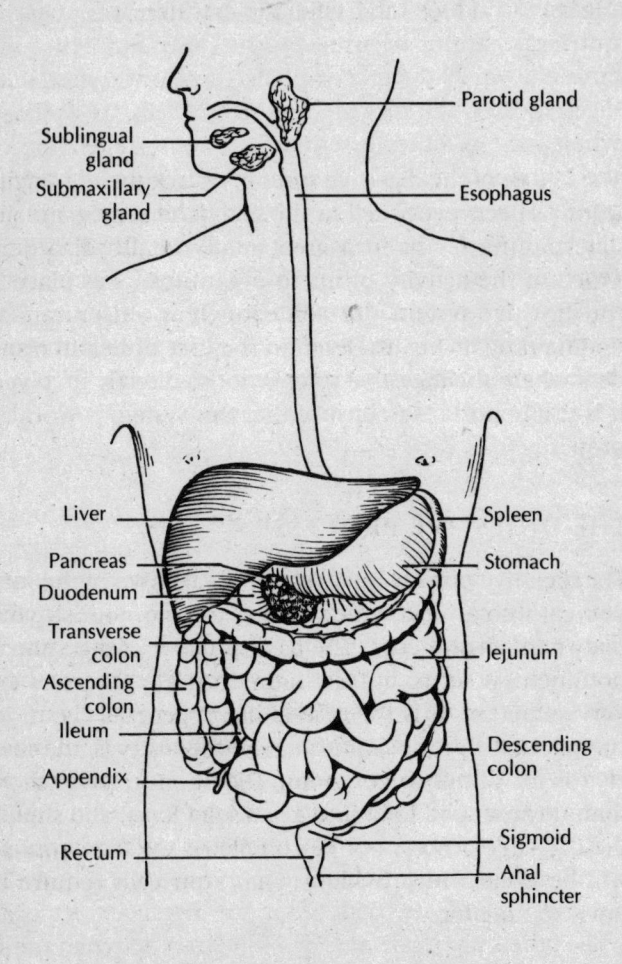

Figure 1: The Digestive System

countless different functions, with the ultimate purpose being to keep you alive. The two classes of nutrients are known as *macronutrients* (which include protein, carbohydrates, and fats) and *micronutrients* (amino acids, simple sugars, fatty acids, and vitamins and minerals). Macronutrients cannot be used by the body until they are broken down by the process of digestion. Once successfully digested they can provide fuel to the cells, as well as a whole host of other essential functions, depending on the nutrient involved. The complete digestion of proteins produces single amino acids of which the protein is actually comprised. Carbohydrates are converted into simple sugars. Fats are broken down into fatty acids. Vitamins and minerals are needed for countless functions, and they work with each other, and with other micronutrients, to keep your body alive and working properly.

THE MECHANICS OF DIGESTION

As mentioned, the method in which your body breaks down food into nourishment is rather complicated, and the network involved in facilitating these digestive processes is equally complex. To give you a point of reference, Figure 1 provides you an outline of the digestive system.

At first glance it may seem inconceivable that all these parts are active in the digestion of food, especially as the food you eat does not come into contact with all of them. However, the digestive system really has two aspects: one involves the specific sites in which digestion takes place; the other represents the chemicals which actually do the digesting. Some of the digestive chemicals (known as *digestive enzymes*) are produced in the digestive tract itself, while others are made outside of the tract and then transported to the relevant sites when needed.

The Mouth

Although the mouth is the first site of digestion, digestive processes (i.e. when the mouth 'waters') can be stimulated by the smell or even by the thought of food. Once in the mouth, chewing begins the mechanical breakdown of the food and functions to increase the surface area of the food to be exposed to digestive enzymes. Chewing also triggers the release of digestive enzymes in the mouth and as well as further down the digestive tract. The enzyme *ptyalin* initiates the breakdown of starches (a form of carbohydrates) in the mouth. This first stage of the reduction of starches into simple sugars is continued later by a related enzyme in the small intestine.

The Stomach

The food moves down the oesophagus into the stomach after it is swallowed. It is here that the stomach continues the mechanical breakdown through a sort of churning process which, among other things, helps mix the food particles with the primary stomach acids and enzymes such as *hydrochloric acid (HCL)* and *pepsin*. These agents facilitate the chemical breakdown of proteins. Proteins consist of amino acids groups which link together to form chains. HCL and pepsin break some of these links to form smaller amino acid chains.

Having an ample supply of these stomach acids and enzymes is vital to your health for many reasons. If levels are insufficient at mealtimes, then protein digestion obviously suffers, with negative implications too varied to discuss here. As it turns out, HCL and pepsin deficiencies are unfortunately very favourable to the spread of *Candida albicans*. This will be discussed in greater detail in Chapter 5.

The Intestinal Tract

After food leaves the stomach it enters the intestinal tract. The *small intestine* is the first section of this tract and is comprised of three sub-sections – the *duodenum*, the *jejunum* and the *ileum*. The *large intestine* is comprised of seven sections, beginning with the *caecum*, then followed by the *ascending colon*, *transverse colon* and *descending colon*, and finally the *sigmoid*, *rectum* and *anus*.

THE SMALL INTESTINE

The small intestine is actually over 20 ft (7 m) long in the average adult, but is referred to as 'small' due to its lesser diameter compared to that of the large intestine. When the small intestine receives food from the stomach, it moves the food downward through its three sections by a process known as *intestinal peristalsis*. After leaving the ileum, the food moves into the (approximately 5-ft/1.5-m long) large intestine.

The small intestine is more than just a tunnel through which food can be transported; it is also the means by which life-giving components of what we eat, such as micronutrients and water, are absorbed. Although absorption takes place throughout the intestines, it occurs mostly in the small intestine, the walls of which are porous enough for micronutrients to permeate through into the bloodstream. In order to improve the efficiency of absorption, the walls of the small intestine are lined with millions of tiny finger-like protuberances, called *villi*. These villi substantially increase the total surface area of the small intestine, thus providing significantly greater absorptive tissue.

Duodenum

The duodenum is actually the busiest site of digestive activity, in that substantial protein, carbohydrate and fat breakdown takes place here. The duodenum, which comprises only about one-twentieth the length of the small intestine, does not manufacture major enzymes and other digestive substances; instead it receives them from the *pancreas* (the pancreatic enzymes *protease, amylase* and *lipase*) and the *gall bladder* (in the form of *bile*). The absorption of various micronutrients (especially trace minerals) also takes place in the duodenum.

Protease enzymes (such as *chymotrypsin, trypsin* and *carboxypeptidase*) carry on from HCL and pepsin with the digestion of protein. As it happens, protease not only digests food proteins, but also helps to control the numbers of pathogenic organisms in the gut (*see Chapter 4*). Pancreatic amylase is a relative of the mouth enzyme ptyalin, and as such carries further the breakdown of carbohydrates into simple sugars. Pancreatic lipase is responsible for most of the digestion of dietary fats, following the work of the enzyme *gastric lipase* in the stomach.

Bile is a substance which is needed for both fat breakdown and the absorption of fats and fat-soluble vitamins such as vitamins A, D, E and K. Bile is manufactured by the *liver* and is stored in the gall bladder, from where it is secreted into the duodenum. Aside from the above duties, bile is yet another digestive substance which plays an important part in controlling pathogenic species in the gut.

Jejunum

The primary site of nutrient absorption is the jejunum, the middle section of the small intestine. It is here that amino acids, simple sugars, most vitamins and a limited amount of minerals will make their way into the bloodstream to be processed by the body for countless functions essential to life.

Food digestion occurs in the jejunum as well, but not exclusively due to enzymes. It is here that friendly bacterial micro-organisms which help advance digestion begin to proliferate in very large numbers. The organisms in question are a family of bacteria known as *lactobacilli*, of which the most well-known and most prominent in the small intestine is *Lactobacillus acidophilus*. Among other functions, bacteria such as *L. acidophilus* aid in the further breakdown of carbohydrates in the gut. For instance, *L. acidophilus* manufactures an enzyme called *lactase* which digests *lactose*, the sugar found in milk. Lactobacilli also play a major role in increasing the acidity of the small intestine, which makes the environment less hospitable for pathogenic organisms. This point is vital to the story of candida and will be discussed in more detail throughout the book.

Ileum

The ileum is the last section of the small intestine and is the site of the absorption of dietary fats and the fat-soluble vitamins. The fats you consume will already have been emulsified by bile and digested by lipase in the duodenum, and once in the ileum they, along with the fat-soluble vitamins, will be carried through the walls along with most of the bile. The ileum and the first section of the large intestine (the caecum) are separated by the *ileocaecal valve*.

The digestive actions of friendly lactobacilli continue in the ileum. Further down this section of the small intestine, the bacterial populations of the lactobacilli and of the *bifidobacteria* (the bacteria most prevalent in the large intestine) blend together to continue their digestive work.

LARGE INTESTINE

As much of the water contained in the intestinal contents has already been absorbed in the small intestine, digested food is more solid by the time it reaches the caecum. The relatively short length of the large intestine and smaller surface area compared to the small intestine only allows for absorption of water and a small amount of micronutrients. Fortunately, by this time most nutrients have already been extracted. Though absorption is minimal, digestion and control of unfriendly organisms is still being carried out by bacteria, primarily bifidobacteria. *Bifidobacterium bifidum* is the main type in this area, and as you will see in Chapter 9 this is a major player in the fight against the overgrowth of *Candida albicans*.

This outline should give you a very basic idea of the process of digestion and, most importantly here, the function of the different parts of the digestive system. Although this book is not specifically about the digestive system, understanding its workings is vital to understanding how candida overgrows and spreads beyond its boundaries in the first place. In addition, inadvertent damage to the intestines leads directly to some of the most prominent symptoms of candidiasis, and indirectly to several of the health disorders which are known to be linked, at least in part, to candida overgrowth.

With the aid of the information in this chapter you will later learn (a) how digestive insufficiency can allow candida problems to occur, (b) how candida-related intestinal damage is linked to disease patterns, (c) how to help improve digestive activity and repair candida-induced damage to the intestinal tract, and (d) how to prevent the spread of candida beyond its normal intestinal environment.

Should significant amounts of candida escape the

confines of the digestive system into the bloodstream, the immune system will become your only defence against the proliferation. The next chapter provides a basic picture of the immune system, to help you to understand how to strengthen its ability to fight candidiasis.

CHAPTER 3

The Immune System

For every second of every day your system is bombarded by potentially damaging influences such as viruses, bacteria, developing cancer cells, and so on; yet, most of the time, you remain free of any acute manifestation of their presence. The reason for this is that you are supplied with a built-in army designed to protect you from anything which does not belong in your body. This army is the immune system. It represents one of the most fascinating and diverse aspects of human biochemistry, and though far too intricate and detailed to cover in its entirety here, a basic outline will help you understand the discussion of candidiasis later in this book.

MAJOR IMMUNE SYSTEM COMPONENTS

The immune system is made up of many different elements, the primary ones being *white blood cells*, lymphatic components such as the *thymus gland* and the *spleen, antibodies*, and various immune hormones and proteins. The *liver* also plays a very important part in immunity. There are other secondary elements as well, but the above are the ones we will focus on here.

White Blood Cells
The main fighting force against infection and cancer are

white blood cells. There are many different types of these cells, each playing its own distinct role in the protection of the body.

The two main types of white blood cells are *T-cells* and *B-cells*. T-cells are made in the thymus gland (*see below*) and are responsible for regulating and directing a great deal of the immune activity which goes on in the body. For example, *T-helper cells* aid in the function of other white blood cells, while *T-suppressor* cells inhibit or moderate such activity. A third type, *cytotoxic T-cells*, directly destroy infected or cancerous cells, among other things. B-cells are made in the bone marrow and produce substances called antibodies (*see below*) which regulate and direct immune activity that is not controlled by T-cells.

Some other types of white blood cells worth mentioning here are *natural killer (NK) cells* and *macrophages*. NK cells destroy infected or damaged cells without having to be directed by T-cells or antibodies, while macrophages devour foreign matter, debris, bacteria and so on.

The Thymus Gland

The thymus gland plays the most diverse role in immune function. This lesser-known gland, which sits behind the breastbone, is the site of T-cell production. Adequate quantities as well as quality of T-cells are essential to a properly functioning immune system. The thymus is also responsible for producing certain hormones needed to activate specific immune processes.

Unfortunately, the thymus gland functions best in childhood, beginning gradually to shrink as you get older. This degeneration can be due to various factors such as damage from free radicals (potentially destructive molecules or molecular fragments), stress, and repeated challenges to the immune system. Even by young adulthood the thymus can be considerably smaller than its original size. Of course, this process is a most unappealing prospect is you suffer with systemic candidiasis and thus have a far greater need for strong T-cell activity (T-cells are especially vital in fighting off fungal challenges to the body). Methods for protecting the thymus and improving its function will be covered in Chapter 9.

Antibodies

In Chapter 1 antibodies were mentioned in reference to certain types of diagnostic test which could be used for determining the presence of candida in the blood. Antibodies are produced by the B-cells in response to certain invaders, such as candida. They bind to the invader, 'memorize' the identity of the invader, and start a chain of events which will ultimately cause other white blood cells to destroy the organism. The role of antibodies in immunity is best illustrated by the concept of vaccinations. In a vaccine you are given minute amounts of what the inoculation is intending to make you immune to. For instance, in a smallpox vaccine you are given a tiny amount of smallpox. The amount used is theoretically not enough to cause harm, but is enough to be recognized by the immune system, thus causing the production of antibodies to initiate its identification and destruction; the point being that if smallpox were to enter your system in larger amounts at a later time, you would already have antibodies set up to deal with it, and the smallpox would be controlled and eliminated from your system before you were properly infected.

The fact that almost everyone has antibodies to candida should theoretically make it easy for the immune system to destroy, but the constant feeding of the blood with a ready-made supply of candida from the digestive tract counteracts this to varying degrees. In order to augment the ability of antibodies to deal with systemic proliferation of candida, the rest of the immune system has to run at full capacity. The problem is that over long periods of overwork, such as is the case with long-term systemic candidiasis, the entire immune system is likely to be considerably weakened; hence the need to boost the immune system and weaken the hold of candida in the digestive system (*see Chapters 8 and 9*).

The Liver

The organ which has the most diverse responsibilities of all is the liver. Although immune function is not its primary purpose, it certainly does play an important role in keeping the body free of harmful invaders. One of the liver's main actions is to filter toxins and foreign invaders from the blood. This detoxification is carried out by certain compounds produced in the liver, as well as by a type of macrophage called *Kupffer cells*. These white blood cells devour foreign substances and certain organisms, including yeasts, very efficiently; enhancing their effects should be a major priority of any candidiasis sufferer.

Actually, improving the overall activity of the liver is a major preventative and therapeutic goal in general. Aside from the direct threat of the candida cells themselves, there is a great increase in the production of toxic substances when candida is prolific. As a matter of fact, the killing of candida itself produces toxic substances which will need to be removed quickly in order to speed recovery and avoid symptoms of 'die off' known as the *Herxheimer reaction*. Methods of accomplishing efficient detoxification and enhancing the activity of macrophages such as the Kupffer cells will be covered in Chapter 9.

The Spleen

The spleen may not be the most well-known organ in the body, but it is vital to efficient immunity from disease. Aside from being a site of production for certain white blood cells involved in destroying harmful organisms, the spleen also produces certain proteins which stimulate immunity.

Many other parts, substances and cells of the body are involved in immune function, but the above represent special priorities for candidiasis sufferers. The next chapter focuses on what is probably of greatest concern to sufferers – the symptoms of candidiasis.

CHAPTER 4

The Common Symptoms
of Candidiasis

At this point it is important to make a distinction between the symptoms of candidiasis and of specific health disorders which are either caused or exacerbated by candida overgrowth. Inevitably there will be some crossover of the two, but in order to give you a clearer picture of things I will for the most part cover the classic symptoms in this chapter and the related disorders in Chapter 7.

There are actually so many symptoms which are typically caused by candidiasis that this has inevitably led to many sufferers being wrongly labelled as hypochondriacs by friends, co-workers, loved ones, and presumably many physicians. Even if not classed as hypochondria, sometimes the whole mess gets put down to stress, emotions, or some other non-specific cause. Doctors are most accustomed to working with individuals who have more classic symptom patterns which match a specific condition. Thanks to doctors like Truss and Crook, many more physicians are becoming aware of candida, but it can take many decades for such revelations to filter through and become accepted by the majority of practising doctors.

As a result, it is not unusual for candidiasis sufferers who are unable to be helped or even properly diagnosed to begin to believe what many have been saying – that the whole problem is in their head. Many others know beyond a shadow of a doubt that something physiological is very wrong, but if unable to find help from the medical profession self-doubt and desperation begin to take hold. This is quite understandable, especially in those cases where the symptoms are so debilitating that sufferers have a difficult time functioning even minimally. There is no set rule for how candidiasis will manifest. In some it will be relatively minor – nagging, but not debilitating. Others will find it difficult even to get out of bed. Still others will fall in the middle or will fluctuate between the two extremes.

COMMON SYMPTOMS

The symptoms of candidiasis vary greatly from person to person, not only in severity but also in the combination of symptoms. It is not unusual for sufferers to develop new symptoms as time goes on. The severity of the symptoms will seldom be static, but instead will fluctuate a great deal depending on various factors such as diet, stress levels, immune function and general environment. The rather substantial list of the most common systems of candidiasis includes:

- headaches
- fatigue
- abdominal bloating
- constipation
- diarrhoea
- gas
- heartburn
- vaginal or oral thrush
- vaginitis
- cystitis
- depression
- anxiety

- irritability
- insomnia
- dizziness or light-headedness
- memory loss
- lack of mental alertness
- skin disorders (e.g. acne)
- allergies (especially to foods)
- sensitivity to chemicals
- menstrual and premenstrual difficulties.

There are also a whole host of health problems which may be triggered by candida infections; these are not symptoms proper, but are rather separate disorders caused or made worse by the spread of candida. This would include among others allergies, chemical sensitivities, chronic fatigue syndrome (ME) and so on. The connection between these conditions and candidiasis will be discussed in Chapter 7. Now we will take a closer look at the above mentioned symptoms.

Digestive Disturbances

One of the primary areas to be thoroughly affected by candida overgrowth is the digestive system. This is perfectly logical considering the fact that this is the primary site of its residence. When candida migrates to other areas of the body, this is not particularly because it finds other parts of the body more hospitable to its presence; quite the contrary. However, when it grows so much in numbers, inevitably its colonies will spread out.

Once the newly created candida cells have so thoroughly dominated their original environment, there will be little opportunity for beneficial strains of bacteria, which are needed for proper digestion and maintenance of a healthy intestinal environment, to survive. In order for the good bacteria to thrive and function, most types need to implant, or settle on the walls of the intestines. If the candida is already using up the available room, then it is difficult for the beneficial types to remain. Aside from this, there is a competition for food. As it happens, both candida and beneficial bacteria thrive on sugars in the gut, and if the lion's share of the available food supply is being hoarded by candida cells, then beneficial bacteria will be eliminated. This accounts for much, though not all, of the explanation for the digestive symptoms such as bloating and gas. These symptoms are typically caused by the production of large amounts of gases such as methane and hydrogen, which are by-products of improper fermentation of incompletely digested foods. This is much more likely to occur when digestive bacteria are at minimal levels, such as in candida overgrowth. The acid reflux which causes heartburn can also be triggered by fermentation gases in the upper digestive tract.

Candida albicans can also negatively influence the peristaltic waves of the intestinal tract, thereby causing either constipation or diarrhoea (or alternation between the two). How it does so will be covered in Chapter 5, but it is worth mentioning here that there is a very close connection between *Candida albicans* infections and irritable bowel syndrome (IBS), which will often manifest with the entire collection of digestive symptoms listed above. The bottom line is that all digestive functions are bound to suffer in the event of intestinal candidiasis.

Emotional and Mental Symptoms

It is true that the stress of having often debilitating physical symptoms can take its toll on you emotionally, manifesting in depression, feelings of helplessness, and so on; however, this is not the only, nor probably even the main cause of the emotional symptoms of candidiasis. One's mood is mediated by a very intricate balance of chemicals in the brain, which appears to be quite easily disturbed by the long-term effects of systemic candidiasis. Brain chemicals accounting for clear thinking, memory, alertness and proper sleep patterns are also affected adversely. Perhaps one of the most likely factors to affect brain function is low blood sugar (hypoglycaemia) which afflicts so many candidiasis sufferers. Lack of mental energy or alertness and deficient memory are classic hypoglycaemia symptoms regardless of the cause. Another manner in which such symptoms can occur is due to chronic malabsorption of nutrients in the intestines, which can be caused by intestinal candida overgrowth. All micronutrients are needed in ample supply for the proper function of the brain and the rest of the central nervous system. If micronutrients are being consumed but are not absorbed into the bloodstream, then brain function suffers, as does the health of the nerves and the rest of the body, for that matter. Especially once systemic, the candida also produces various toxins which can significantly alter normal brain chemistry.

Headaches and Dizziness

Low blood sugar is frequently implicated in the symptoms of headaches and dizziness, especially when they occur in combination. In candidiasis, headaches can also be a side-effect of the significant build-up of toxins which is unavoidable in unchecked candida overgrowth, especially when systemic. This is a very important issue and will be discussed in detail in Chapter 5. With candida-related migraine headaches, chances are that they are being caused by reactions to certain things you are eating. Migraines are often associated with food allergies, as well as increased sensitivity to certain naturally occurring chemicals contained in various food types. Of course, both food allergies and chemical sensitivity are prevalent in candidiasis.

Fatigue

Fatigue is such a non-specific term that it is difficult to ever know its exact origin. There are several likely explanations in candidiasis: energy used up by an over-worked immune system; hypoglycaemia; nutritional deficiencies caused by malabsorption. It is not difficult to imagine how fatigue could be a major symptom of hypoglycaemia, as blood sugar is needed for energy within the brain and throughout the body. Deficiencies caused through malabsorption can impair the conversion of food into energy – a process requiring many micronutrients. When the body's defence force, the immune system, is taxed an enormous amount of energy is used in the process. As you will see in Chapter 5, once candida becomes systemic the immune system will be the only means of controlling it.

Local Thrush Infections

A symptom which is familiar to many is the local thrush infection which occurs most often in the vaginal canal, or less frequently in the mouth or the anus. Thrush infections are due to the rather extreme accumulation of yeast cells in one of the orifices of the body. It is quite normal for candida to reside in areas other than the intestines, such as the vaginal canal in women; however, as with all yeast problems, all it takes is a suitable environment for proliferation and then problems will occur. These events are very often classed generically as 'yeast infections'.

Although this is the most well-recognized candida manifestation, it does not occur in all or even most cases of candidiasis, even of the more severe systemic variety. As a result, you should not assume that candida is in control if there is no visible yeast proliferation. A single thrush infection does not mean that a person has severe candidiasis throughout the body, but if thrush becomes more prevalent, then the likelihood of systemic spread looms ever larger.

Vaginitis and Cystitis

A local yeast infection can also give rise to many other adverse consequences. Vaginitis, an irritation and inflammation of the vaginal tissue, is one such example. When yeast proliferates in the vaginal canal it alters the normal environment of the area, accounting for problems such as irritation, itching and dryness, and often significant pain during sexual intercourse.

Cystitis, which manifests as pain and irritation in the urinary tract, is generally a result of the migration of pathogenic bacteria from other parts of the body into the urinary tract. The type of bacteria which normally account for urinary tract infections (UTIs) find it much easier to proliferate when candida overgrowth weakens the immune system or reduces beneficial bacteria levels in the faeces (where the cystitis bacteria are often derived). Candida itself can cause its fair share of problems in the urinary tract regardless of the damage caused by pathogenic bacteria.

Allergies

The increased likelihood of allergies is not so much a symptom of candidiasis as a separate disorder which can be caused or made worse by candida overgrowth. There are two main factors accounting for increased allergic tendencies. First is the increased absorption of allergic components from food caused by candida damage to the intestinal tract. Second is the generally imbalanced state of the immune system in the presence of systemic candidiasis. This subject will be covered in more detail in Chapter 7.

Skin Disorders

Increased tendency toward acne is a common complaint of those with yeast problems. A strong immune system will prevent acne development by killing the bacteria responsible for the condition, but as you can imagine, this focus is likely to be compromised by the fight to control candida in and around the body. Any malabsorptive tendencies can also make the healing of acne lesions more difficult due to deficiencies in nutrients involved in tissue repair and immune function.

The inflamed patches of *eczema* or *psoriasis* are not at all uncommon. Eczema is most heavily linked to food allergies and the overgrowth of *staphylococcus aureas* bacteria. Psoriasis is typically manifested in inflamed skin patches on which skin cells pile up, forming scales. This is associated with a defect in the skin cells which can be caused by intestinally-derived toxins which can build up, especially in the presence of candida overgrowth. The liver would normally neutralize these toxins before they caused too many problems, but in candidiasis the liver is generally overworked trying to deal with candida-derived toxins.

Menstrual and Premenstrual Difficulties

The hormone imbalances which can be triggered by candidiasis are a perfect example of how candida can either directly or indirectly affect the entire functioning of the body. There are so many possible explanations for an increased tendency for hormone imbalances that it is impossible to know which, if any, is more important than the others. General malfunction of the endocrine system, influences on brain chemistry, yeast overgrowth in the reproductive cavity, hypoglycaemia, malabsorption and many other explanations are possible.

No matter how the candidiasis expresses itself, it will often appear better or worse depending on the environment. For instance, it is very common for symptoms to heighten when it is damp or muggy. Not surprisingly, it is also common for an exacerbation of symptoms to occur when you are exposed to places infested with mould, such as a damp, dark area (basements, storage rooms, etc.). As a result, it is highly recommended to avoid such environments and contact with mouldy objects (such as old books or clothing stored in cool, dark storage closets, etc.) as much as possible until you have adequately recovered.

The above symptoms represent the most common manifestations of candidiasis, although there are still others that are associated with this condition. Suffice it to say that, if candidiasis is the cause, when the overgrowth is effectively treated and reversed such symptoms should either improve significantly or disappear completely.

CHAPTER 5

The Causes of Candidiasis

It is understandable that most of the focus of candidiasis sufferers will be on symptoms, but these are actually more helpful for diagnosing the condition than for treating it. Among other things, the prospect of treating several symptoms (often related to different systems in the body) at once is not realistic. Candidiasis is unique in its control over the body and often symptomatic treatments do not work particularly well if the candida itself is not being addressed. Even if symptomatic treatment were more appropriate and effective, if the underlying causes are not addressed then symptomatic treatments may become a permanent requirement. Of course, a successful treatment of the cause or causes will eventually, if not immediately, improve the symptoms anyway. Once you know that candidiasis is the cause of your symptoms, the next step is to discover what causes the candida to get out of control in the first place.

BACTERIAL IMBALANCE

As you know, the difference between a person who suffers with candidiasis and one who does not is that the sufferer is no longer able to keep the candida in controlled numbers and isolated in its normal habitat. As it is primarily the beneficial bacteria in the body which exert this control, the first thing which must take place for candida to get out of hand is for these bacteria to be insufficient to carry out this task. There are really many things which can alter the numbers of friendly organisms such as *lactobacilli* and *bifidobacteria*; the use of prescription antibiotics being the classic example (*see page 34*).

REDUCED DIGESTIVE SECRETIONS

As you will recall from Chapter 2, various digestive secretions play a secondary role in the control of organisms such as yeasts, harmful bacteria, protozoa, worms, etc. There are many different digestive substances which perform this task, the most important being the protease enzymes secreted by the pancreas, stomach enzymes such as hydrochloric acid (HCL) and pepsin, and bile (which is produced by the liver). These substances help control candida spread especially in the upper digestive tract, boosting the action of the beneficial bacteria. The efficient production and/or release of digestive substances is prone to impairment by various influences (*see pages 36–8*).

IMMUNE SYSTEM WEAKNESS

As the immune system represents your body's main defence against infection by pathogenic organisms such as *Candida albicans*, it is undeniable that any weakness in its function can facilitate the proliferation of candida in the blood and body tissues. The candida – immune system connection results in a particularly vicious circle. You will recall that the main gland of immunity, the thymus, is weakened by overwork during infection. Systemic yeast/fungus proliferation is an infection that requires constant hyperactivity of the immune system, thereby weakening immunity further, which allows the yeast to proliferate even more, and so on. Regardless of the direct effect of infections on the thymus, if the white blood cells are having to donate so much of their efforts to dealing with candida in the blood and tissues, then they will not be as efficient in dealing with viruses, harmful bacteria, etc. Aside from the candida itself, there are many outside influences which can substantially compromise immune response.

FEEDING THE YEAST

As *Candida albicans* is a living organism, it must have a source of sustenance to survive. Its preferred form of food is sugar, which it will readily take from the body and use to facilitate the growth of its colonies. Although this point will be elucidated in detail in Chapter 8, its importance deserves repeated emphasis, especially as it is one of the factors of candidiasis which is most readily within your control. The extent to which you avoid inadvertently feeding candida is pivotal if you are to reverse candidiasis and ultimately eliminate its symptoms.

Some of the major influences which adversely alter digestive bacterial balance, digestive secretions and immune function, and which generally favour yeast proliferation, include antibiotics, antacids, steroids, oral contraceptives, stress, and diet.

Antibiotics

The rather liberal use of antibiotics in Western countries has undoubtedly done much to perpetuate the ever-increasing numbers of candidiasis sufferers. Antibiotics are used for treating not only major infections but also (and far too frequently) minor ones as well. Another common practice is to use them in therapy for acne. Whatever the reason, prescription antibiotics (especially if used for extended periods and/or on multiple occasions) is thought to be the most common cause of candidiasis.

The main problem with antibiotics stems from the fact that while they are prescribed with the intent to kill whatever pathogenic bacteria are infecting you, they inadvertently kill the beneficial type at the same time. Very simply put, the numbers of lactobacilli and bifidobacteria are substantially reduced or, with long-term or repeated use, decimated. As you would expect, this allows candida cells to multiply and colonies to spread unchecked. It might be slightly different if prescribed antibiotics were also able to kill fungi, but this is not the case. Oddly enough, it used to be common practice to prescribe fungus-killing drugs when antibiotics were being employed, but this is not typically the case today. In addition to killing protective bacteria, prescribed antibiotics can have a detrimental effect on immune function.

There are times, such as in very severe infections, when strong antibiotics can save lives, so it is not being suggested that they never be used. It is just that there are many occasions when they are not necessary or even helpful for what they are being prescribed. It is interesting to note that, not long before the time of writing, the British Minister of Health went on record saying that antibiotics were often being used inappropriately, and beseeched doctors to be more judicious in prescribing them. At any rate, regardless of how and why they are being used, it would make all the difference in the world if it became common practice to replace (preferably through supplements) the lactobacilli and bifidobacteria that are destroyed by antibiotics. Some of the more progressive doctors already make this recommendation to their patients, but they are a very small minority. The use and benefits of such supplements will be discussed in depth in Chapter 9.

Antacids

Among the most heavily prescribed drugs in the world are those used for the treatment of excess acid in the stomach. Less powerful forms of these medicines are also very popular over-the-counter (OTC). Most prescriptions are written for the type of antacids which inhibit the release of digestive acids such as hydrochloric acid (HCL) in the stomach. This type is often used for the treatment of ulcers. Others, and especially the OTC forms, often work by neutralizing acid in the stomach after it has been released. These are commonly selected by those who experience acid indigestion and heartburn following meals.

Because these drugs impair the release or activity of digestive acids, the important defence digestive secretions provide against candida and other organisms in the upper digestive tract can be damaged to varying degrees. The extent of this impairment will depend on the type, quantity and frequency of the medication, as well as the sufferer's unique biochemistry. It is interesting to note that heartburn and acid indigestion are often a symptom of *too little* acid being released into the stomach when food is eaten. This can cause fermentation by-products such as gases, which lead to gastric reflux (flushing of acid from the stomach back into the oesophagus) and its above-mentioned manifestations. As a result, many of those who use OTC medicines for neutralizing acid stomach may risk exacerbating not only candidiasis but any indigestion problem, in spite of lessening temporarily their symptoms. There are people who really do produce too much stomach acid at the wrong time, so you should not stop using any such medication without getting consent from a qualified health practitioner, especially if you have a history of stomach ulcers. Having said this, there seem to be significant limitations to the benefits of acid-blocking or neutralizing medications in many cases, and they are generally over-used.

Steroids

Drugs from the *corticosteroid* category (such as cortisone) are also infamous for their ability to perpetuate candidiasis. In this case it is not so much their effect on candida in the intestines but rather the proliferation in the bloodstream and tissues. Corticosteroids, often called 'steroids', are occasionally prescribed either for their significant anti-inflammatory effect (as in asthma treatment) or as an immune suppressant (as in auto-immune disorders such as rheumatoid arthritis). Doctors are aware of the long list of significant side-effects from steroid use, especially when ingested, but their ability to perpetuate systemic candidiasis is seldom acknowledged.

With respect to candida, the destructiveness of steroids is pretty straightforward. Due to their substantial suppressant effect on the immune system, steroids inhibit the defence force which can kill the candida systemically.

Oral Contraceptives

The contraceptive pill has also been implicated as a common contributor to candida overgrowth. The prevalence of candida overgrowth in the vaginal cavity is alarmingly high in women using the Pill. In his book *The Missing Diagnosis*, C. Orian Truss M.D. suggests that the progesterone constituents of various oral contraceptives may be the crux of the problem; this is based on his observation that vaginal yeast irritation is at its worst when a woman's progesterone levels are elevated. William Crook M.D. in his book *The Yeast Connection* states that such yeast over-growth is thought to be due to changes in the vaginal mucosal tissue. He goes on to point out that oestrogen-only preparations often prescribed for menopausal or post-menopausal women do not appear to encourage candida growth.

Stress

Simply put, stress is any factor – whether emotional, mental, physical or environmental – that alters the normal function of the body. Stress affects digestive secretions considerably. Thus difficulties at work, arguments at home, worries about financial issues, being in a hurry, excessive physical activity, lack of sleep, etc. – to mention just a few of the many stresses in our lives – can challenge the efficiency of our digestive processes.

From the standpoint of digestion, stress in and of itself is not really the problem; it is rather the hormonal reactions brought about by the body in response to stress. Certain hormones which are released by the adrenal glands during stress shunt blood circulation away from the digestive system and direct it to other parts of the body. This process inhibits the release of digestive substances into the stomach and intestines, thereby reducing digestive strength. This is often why we get indigestion if we eat when we are highly stressed. Of course, this effect on digestive release also would reduce the control of pathogenic organisms in the gut.

Another way in which stress poses problems to the candidiasis sufferer is through its effects on the immune system. As you know, adrenal steroids are sometimes used as medication with the intention of suppressing the immune system. These steroids are pharmaceutically produced forms of the steroids which your body releases when under stress; therefore, not surprisingly, stress (especially when chronic) will have immune-suppressive effects as well.

Diet

There are so many aspects of diet which can contribute to an increased risk or worsening of candidiasis. Dietary mismanagement can adversely affect bacterial balance, digestive secretions and immune function. It can also be a significant factor in your tolerance (or lack thereof) to stress. Also very important to the development, or conversely the treatment of candidiasis, your diet helps determine whether or not the candida has a readily available and plentiful food supply on which to feed and proliferate.

Where candidiasis is concerned, dietary management is not so much an issue of how much you eat, rather of *what* you eat (or drink). Though your diet influences your state of health whether you suffer with yeast overgrowth or not, candidiasis is one of the best examples of a condition which can be significantly worsened even by certain very 'healthy' foods. The clinical observations of practitioners who have treated candidiasis over the years provide the best evidence of the dietary approach most likely to be successful for controlling and/or treating it. The type and duration of such changes will vary from person to person, but there are some general rules that apply to the majority of sufferers. Changing your diet is for many people a most unappealing affair, but considering its huge role in treatment and recovery it is well worth the effort. For a complete discussion of dietary influences on candidiasis, please see Chapter 8.

CHAPTER 6

Candida Questionnaire

Now that you are familiar with the typical symptom patterns and the factors most likely to cause candidiasis, it is recommended that you apply this information to your own situation by filling in a 'candida questionnaire'. The optimal approach in diagnosing candidiasis would involve the questionnaire being corroborated by blood antibody testing and/or stool culture testing. Even without the lab tests, a well-designed questionnaire is invaluable in helping you or your healthcare practitioner determine whether any of your symptoms or health problems are connected with candidiasis; this is especially important when you consider the limitations of lab testing for candida (as mentioned in Chapter 1).

An excellent and very comprehensive candida questionnaire was developed by one of the pioneers in candida awareness, William Crook M.D. The questionnaire used here is from Dr Crook's best-selling book *The Yeast Connection*.

CANDIDA QUESTIONNAIRE AND SCORE SHEET

Section A: History

Circle the score for each question to which you answer 'yes', then add up the scores for each 'yes' answer and record it at the bottom of this section.

1 Have you taken tetracyclines or any other antibiotics for acne for one month or longer?   35

2 Have you, at any time in your life, taken other 'broad-spectrum' antibiotics for respiratory, urinary or other infections (for two months or longer, or in shorter courses four or more times in a one-year period?   35

3 Have you taken a broad-spectrum antibiotic drug – even a single course?   6

4 Have you, at any time in your life, been bothered by persistent prostatitis, vaginitis or other problems affecting your reproductive organs?   25

5 Have you been pregnant two or more times?   5

5a One time?   3

6 Have you taken birth control pills for more than two years?   15

6a For six months to two years?   8

7 Have you taken prednisone or other cortisone-type drugs for more than two weeks?   15

7a For two weeks or less?   6

8 Does exposure to perfumes, insecticides, fabric shop odours and other chemicals provoke *moderate to severe* symptoms?   20

8a *Mild* symptoms?   5

9 Are your symptoms worse on damp, muggy days or in mouldy places?   20

10 Have you had athlete's foot, ring worm, or other fungus infections of the skin or nails? If so, have such infections been *severe or persistent*?   20

10a *Mild to moderate*?	10
11 Do you crave sugar?	10
12 Do you crave breads?	10
13 Do you crave alcoholic beverages?	10
14 Does tobacco smoke really bother you?	10

Total Score Section A: _____

Section B: Major Symptoms

For each of your symptoms, note down the appropriate figure:

    If a symptom is *occasional or mild* – 3

    If a symptom is *frequent and/or moderately severe* – 6

    If a symptom is *severe and/or disabling* – 9

Add up your total score and record it at the bottom of this section.

Fatigue or lethargy	_____
Feeling of being 'drained'	_____
Depression	_____
Poor memory	_____
Feeling 'spacey' or 'unreal'	_____
Inability to make decisions	_____
Numbness, burning or tingling	_____
Headache	_____
Muscle aches	_____
Muscle weakness or paralysis	_____
Pain and/or swelling in joints	_____
Abdominal pain	_____
Constipation and/or diarrhoea	_____
Bloating, belching or intestinal gas	_____
Troublesome vaginal burning, itching or discharge	_____
Prostatitis	_____
Impotence	_____
Loss of sexual desire or feeling	_____
Endometriosis or infertility	_____
Cramps and/or other menstrual irregularities	_____

Premenstrual tension ____

Attacks of anxiety and crying ____

Cold hands or feet and/or chilliness ____

Shaking or irritable when hungry ____

Total Score Section B: ____

Section C: Other Symptoms

For each of your symptoms, note down the appropriate figure:

If a symptom is *occasional or mild* – 1

If a symptom is *frequent and/or moderately severe* – 2

If a symptom is *severe and/or disabling* – 3

Add up your total score and record it at the bottom of this section.

Drowsiness ____

Irritability or jitteriness ____

Lack of coordination ____

Inability to concentrate ____

Frequent mood swings ____

Insomnia ____

Dizziness/loss of balance ____

Pressure above ears ... feeling of head swelling ____

Tendency to bruise easily ____

Chronic rashes or itching ____

Numbness, tingling ____

Indigestion or heartburn ____

Food sensitivity or intolerance ____

Mucus in stools ____

Rectal itching ____

Dry mouth or throat ____

Rash or blisters in mouth ____

Bad breath ____

Foot, hair or body odour not relieved by washing ____

Nasal congestion or post-nasal drip   _____

Nasal itching   _____

Sore throat   _____

Laryngitis, loss of voice   _____

Cough or recurrent bronchitis   _____

Pain or tightness in chest   _____

Wheezing or shortness of breath   _____

Urinary frequency or urgency   _____

Burning on urination   _____

Spots in front of eyes or erratic vision   _____

Burning or tearing of eyes   _____

Recurrent infections or fluid in the ears   _____

Ear pain or deafness   _____

Total Score Section C: _____

GRAND TOTAL: _____

The grand total score will help you and your physician decide if your health problems are yeast-connected.

(Scores in women will run higher, as five questions in the questionnaire apply exclusively to women, while only two apply exclusively to men.)

Assessing Your Score

The final part of this questionnaire will give you an idea of the likelihood of candidiasis based on your final score[1].

Over 180 (women)/140 (men):
Yeast-connected health problems are almost certainly present.

Over 120 (women)/90 (men):
Yeast-connected health problems are probably present.

Over 60 (women)/40 (men):
Yeast-connected health problems are possibly present.

Less than 60 (women)/40 (men):
Yeasts are probably not causing your health problems.

[1] From William G. Crook M.D., *The Yeast Connection* (Jackson, TN: Professional Books; New York: Vintage Books, 3rd edn, 1986) and *The Yeast Connection and the Woman* (Jackson, TN: Professional Books, 1995).

CHAPTER 7

Other Disorders Associated with Candidiasis

Hopefully the previous chapters have given you a clearer picture of the way in which candidiasis typically develops and manifests. Now we shall look at some of the health problems that can either be caused or significantly affected by candidiasis. When systemic, candidiasis can be a factor in more or less all health problems. The following represent some of the most heavily researched and clinically reported examples.

MYALGIC ENCEPHALOMYELITIS (ME)

This disorder, which is often referred to as *chronic fatigue syndrome*, is a classic example of a condition which typically has candidiasis as an associated problem. Chronic fatigue is the main symptom of ME, although as with systemic candidiasis there are a great many other associated symptoms. It is interesting that the orthodox medical profession has shown some resistance to recognizing ME as a 'real' disorder, just as it has resisted recognizing candidiasis. Again, this resistance is beginning to weaken (albeit slowly), due to the fact that research has confirmed that the cause of ME is physiological and not purely psychosomatic, as many cynics have suggested.

There are so many symptoms in common between the two disorders that one could not help but to suspect a link.

As it turns out, people who are properly diagnosed as suffering with ME frequently have a significant problem with systemic candida overgrowth. Such an association would not necessarily guarantee a tangible link in all people, but what is obvious is that in both cases the immune system is inextricably involved. As you know, a weakness in the immune system allows candida to proliferate systemically. Such proliferation weakens the immune system even further. The same vicious circle applies to ME, which is associated with the unchecked spread of certain viruses (such as Epstein Barr, cytomegalovirus, etc.). Immune weakness caused by systemic candidiasis keeps the body from controlling ME-related viruses, and vice versa – which develops first will depend on the individual.

The main importance of the association is that by successfully treating one, you are likely to improve the other significantly. A typical natural approach to treating ME would be to strengthen the immune system to control the viruses. However, unlike ME, candida in the blood and tissues can constantly be added to by a flourishing supply in the gut. This requires that treatment take into account strengthening the immune system *and* stemming the gut proliferation. As a result, if both disorders are present a comprehensive systemic candidiasis treatment is liable to benefit both conditions more than would treating the ME alone (i.e. through immune stimulation).

ALLERGIES

It is common to refer to an allergy as an abnormal sensitivity to a substance which produces an adverse reaction. Technically speaking this is not the complete definition, as you can have an abnormal reaction to a substance which is not allergic in nature. In an allergy the sensitivity and subsequent reaction are mediated by a specialized response from your immune system. In processes which are similar though slightly different than those which involve viruses, bacteria, etc., the immune system recognizes and attacks certain components which gain entry into the bloodstream, thereby setting up a chain of events culminating in the adverse symptom. Attacks of allergens involve special types of antibodies, which as you may recall bind to the invader and trigger their destruction by certain white blood cells. The first stage of an allergy will be the absorption of the allergic substance, typically some type of protein, into the bloodstream. Fortunately the body has certain defences designed to prevent the absorption of allergic proteins in the first place.

Food Allergies

The defence mechanism in the case of food allergies is twofold. The foods you eat are supposed to be broken down by the process of digestion into their most basic components. For example, proteins are broken down into amino acids, carbohydrates into simple sugars, and fats into fatty acids. Along with vitamins and minerals, amino acids, simple sugars, and fatty acids are referred to as *micronutrients*. Interestingly, while large proteins are detected and attacked, amino acids are not considered invaders by the body. As a result, the first defence against allergies is to ensure complete breakdown of dietary protein into its amino acid components. If this is accomplished then there is no chance of an allergic reaction to any proteins that have been eaten.

Unfortunately, it is not unusual for some food proteins in a meal to be incompletely digested. Even in this case, however, the body has 'a second line of defence': the intestinal wall, through which almost all food components are absorbed. This wall is designed to be only just permeable enough to allow micronutrients and water to pass through it. Like the fine mesh of a coffee filter, the healthy intestinal wall will keep out large molecules such as undigested food proteins.

Excessive Intestinal Permeability and Bowel Toxins

Unfortunately, in some people the permeability of the intestinal wall is such that larger proteins are allowed to pass through. This condition, sometimes referred to as 'leaky gut', is caused by a breakdown of the connective tissue which provides integrity to the intestinal mucous membrane. There can be various causes for this loss of integrity, including intestinally-produced toxins, nutritional deficiencies, damage from free radicals (highly reactive molecules or molecular fragments), and the activity of the mycelial form of candida.

When candida converts into its mycelial fungal form it can penetrate the intestinal mucosal cells. Candida is also notorious for its toxic by-products, which can damage the gut wall. Aside from its own toxic by-products, by competing with beneficial bacteria in the gut *Candida albicans* can allow toxins from pathogenic bacteria to abound as well. One particularly destructive class of such toxins are called *polyamines*. These are produced when certain bacteria break down incompletely digested proteins in the intestines. Absorbed polyamines have also been linked to the skin disorder *psoriasis*, and to certain forms of arthritis. Yet another potential way in which candida can affect intestinal integrity is through allergic mechanisms. Yeast allergies are common in candidiasis sufferers, and immune-mediated reactions to yeast cells in the intestinal lining can further irritate the mucosa. All this ultimately leads to an increased absorption of any undigested food proteins, and thus an increased propensity to food allergies. Allergies to foods can be experienced in any part of the body, with a wide array of possible symptoms.

Other Allergies

The subject of tissue permeability also applies to other mucous membranes, such as that of the respiratory tract. For instance, candida overgrowth can adversely affect the integrity of the lung and upper respiratory system, thereby increasing their sensitivity to inhaled allergens such as pollens, grasses, dust, mould spores, animal dander and so on. When the proteins from these potential allergens reach the weakened and hypersensitive respiratory walls, the end results are the all-too-common symptoms of sneezing, runny nose, itching and so on. Candida infiltration of this tract also can lead to increased likelihood of respiratory reactions to foods – catarrh build-up being one such reaction. Although not so much allergy-related, candidiasis sufferers are often irritated by cigarette smoke much more than the average person.

CHEMICAL SENSITIVITIES

Another interesting yet distressing feature of systemic candidiasis is the sufferer's reduced tolerance to many chemicals. The list of chemicals which seem to be problematic is vast, but some of the more common include cleaning solvents, paint fumes, synthetic dyes (for example those used in some carpets and clothing), perfume and so on. Actually, everyone is intolerant to industrial chemicals at a certain level; the difference in candidiasis sufferers is that the sensitivity typically manifests after even very slight exposure.

Decreased liver functioning is the link between candida

and increased chemical sensitivity. The liver is responsible for filtering any chemicals and agents (particularly those produced by free radicals) which may otherwise build up and cause a toxic reaction. A healthy liver produces very powerful *antioxidants* which neutralize these free radicals. The liver of a person with candidiasis, however, will not be able to function effectively as it will already be overworked trying to remove candida-derived toxins and those produced by pathogenic bacteria.

Many essential vitamins, minerals, dietary amino acids and herbal constituents also act as antioxidants and may aid in reducing such harmful reactions. Some of these will be discussed in Chapter 9.

IRRITABLE BOWEL SYNDROME (IBS) AND OTHER INTESTINAL DISORDERS

It is thought that up to half of all referrals to gastroenterologists are due to the non-specific intestinal disorder known as Irritable Bowel Syndrome (IBS). This condition is due to a malfunction in the colon (large intestine), resulting in digestive symptoms such as chronic diarrhoea, constipation, abdominal bloating, gas, nausea, lack of appetite and passing of mucus in the stool. It is common for sufferers to experience repeated spasms of the colonic muscle, which cause either diarrhoea or conversely a temporary alteration of the intestinal peristalsis leading to constipation.

About half of all cases of IBS have been linked to food sensitivities of one sort or another, and due to the area affected and the nature of the symptoms there is likely to be a yeast correlation in many cases. IBS does not appear to involve a structural defect, nor does it involve severe inflammation of the colon. It is not a disease *per se*, but rather a non-specific complex of related symptoms. Because of this, diagnosis is primarily made by analysing the symptoms of the person and ruling out other more specific medical disorders such as inflammatory bowel disease (*see below*), diverticular disease, coeliac disease, etc. Many, and sometimes all of the common symptoms of IBS occur in people with intestinal candidiasis. While not all IBS sufferers will necessarily have intestinal candidiasis, over time severe intestinal candidiasis will almost certainly lead to what could be generically classed as IBS.

Inflammatory Bowel Disease (IBD)

In spite of its very distressing symptoms, IBS is among the less severe bowel dysfunctions. There is a class of diseases collectively referred to as IBD which can be quite serious and debilitating. *Ulcerative colitis* and *Crohn's disease* are members of this group and involve significant inflammation of the intestinal tissue and bleeding from the bowel.

These conditions belong to a category of diseases called *auto-immune disorders* which also includes rheumatoid arthritis, multiple sclerosis (MS) and lupus erythematosus, among others. The term 'auto-immune' means that the immune system mistakenly attacks certain tissues of the body. In the case of IBD, the tissues that are attacked are in the intestinal tract.

As you can probably imagine, something goes very wrong in order to allow this to occur. Such cases of 'mistaken identity' are more likely when the tissues are over-run with invaders and thus with circulating antibodies and attacking white blood cells. It is conceivable that such hyperactivity of the immune system along the intestinal wall could accidentally trigger an attack on healthy gut tissue (the gut cells being identified as 'invaders' by antibodies). While it is not certain whether intestinal candidiasis ever actually *causes* IBD (though this is possible), it can certainly exacerbate the condition once IBD exists.

PSYCHOLOGICAL DISORDERS

In spite of the fact that candidiasis is a physiological disorder, this is not to say that it has no affect on the mind or emotions; most who develop systemic candidiasis complain of various psychological problems such as depression, lack of self-esteem, anxiety and excessive worry, apathy, hopelessness and even, in extreme cases, suicidal tendencies. As mentioned earlier, candida-toxins, low blood sugar, hormone imbalance and other physiological features of systemic proliferation can adversely influence brain chemistry, thus accounting for at least some of the psychological symptoms. Aside from these factors, by nature candidiasis is quite a stressful condition in and of itself. When candidiasis is chronic, this would make any feelings of helplessness and desperation understandable. Fortunately, there is ever-growing research which shows that this condition can be successfully treated, and the next two chapters are dedicated to this information.

ACETALDEHYDE

One of the more fascinating correlations between yeast-related toxins and candidiasis symptoms is that of the production of *acetaldehyde*. Acetaldehyde is better known for being the toxin produced from alcohol metabolism in the liver. As a matter of fact, it is primarily acetaldehyde poisoning which is associated with hangovers. The production of acetaldehyde in candidiasis is indirectly caused by the fermentation of sugars in the body by yeast.

It is interesting to note that there are documented cases of people who have been legally drunk although they have not consumed even a drop of alcohol. As you can probably imagine, the possibility of 'auto-intoxication' was met with curious interest by the medical community. Eventually the discovery was made that the source of the alcohol production was indeed internal. It has been reported that a very severe proliferation of candida can produce substantial amounts of alcohol as a by-product of the sugar-fermenting ability of candida. This appears to cause all the classic symptoms of drunkenness in some people. When the internally-produced alcohol is processed in the liver, acetaldehyde is produced – hence the 'hangover' feeling.

This discovery was made many years ago, but it is not as unusual as you might think. Candida, given the right opportunity, can make enough alcohol to produce at least minimal symptoms such as 'spaciness' or difficulty in focusing mentally. Seldom will this produce actual intoxication, but the possibility makes it even more important to avoid sugar strictly in the initial stages of any candidiasis treatment.

PART 2

Treating Candidiasis

CHAPTER 8

Candida Control Diet

The first priority in gaining control over this parasitic yeast/fungus is to be aware of what allows it to thrive and proliferate. The first step is to take a long, hard look at the way you eat. Once you know how to manipulate your diet to avoid yeast overgrowth, you can then look towards methods of killing the candida outright. It is also important to repair the damage to your body caused by the candida infection, and to prevent it from taking over again in the future. Along with this diet, a more proactive approach utilizing nutritional and herbal supplementation is outlined in Chapter 9. Please note that the dietary restrictions discussed in this chapter are not a casual recommendation. The fastest possible recovery unquestionably relies on just how well you follow the information given here.

Although there are some recommendations which will be universally appropriate, because candida can affect the entire body in so many different ways you may need to make slight adjustments to get the best results. As far as the universal recommendations are concerned, effective control and treatment of candidiasis does not lend itself to much flexibility. This dilemma stems from the fact that candidiasis is not a degenerative disorder which gets worse in a predictably gradual pattern, such as arthritis or heart disease; *Candida albicans* is a pathogenic parasite with a voracious appetite and potentially prolific rate of reproduction. In its mycelial fungal form it is a tiny monster with significant territorial objectives and very few limitations.

In spite of the undeniable scope of the fungal form of candida, there are a few distinct advantages in the battle against it. Candida is genetically programmed to do what it does, while you, the sufferer, can think and choose and make adjustments in your approach. You also have the 'advantage' that your symptoms give you – a motivation to do most anything in your power to defeat these freeloading little beasts. Your third advantage is the information in this book – information based on published medical and scientific research and the substantial experience of many clinicians who treat candidiasis on a daily basis – which will allow you to succeed as quickly as possible.

Qualified practitioners are becoming more or less unanimous in their use of dietary manipulation to treat systemic candidiasis. It is not that this is the only approach used – far from it; it is just that candida overgrowth and, conversely, candida control is universally affected by what we eat. Although many people would prefer to 'pop a pill' rather than change their diet, the need to follow the information in this chapter cannot be overemphasized. It is at this impasse that you should use your second advantage over the candida to maintain your commitment to the programme – *motivation*. Candidiasis is often so chronically debilitating that the prospect of being free of it is often enough to make even the most reticent of sufferers consider the effort worthwhile.

Some of the following information should be followed very strictly, especially in the initial stages of the candida control programme. Other recommendations are not as pivotal, but following them as best as possible will certainly aid in the speed of recovery, strengthening of the immune system, repair of weakened body tissues and so on.

Simply put, if you want to get rid of any organism, whether big or small, strong or weak, visible or invisible, the most certain way is to take away its food supply – literally to starve it to death. The first step, therefore, is to stop feeding the yeast.

SUGAR

This is probably not the first time you have been warned away from sugar, and it will probably not be the last. You may be surprised, however, by some of the reasons why it is especially destructive to anyone suffering with candidiasis. Sugar is an interesting paradox in that it provides energy to our cells, which keeps us alive, and yet it can harm our bodies in so many different ways if eaten in excess of our requirements. The answer to this dilemma is that sugar comes in different forms, some of which do not cause the typical problems associated with sugar.

Simple vs. Complex Carbohydrates

Sugars are the basic components of *carbohydrates* in the foods you eat, and serve as a primary energy source for your body. Carbohydrates come in two forms within foods – *simple* and *complex*. Knowing the difference between the two will help you to choose which forms to eat and which to avoid in order to deny candida its sustenance.

Some examples of simple carbohydrates and sweeteners containing them include:

- white table sugar (sucrose)
- brown sugar
- honey

- glucose
- fructose/levulose (fruit sugars)
- fruits and fruit juices
- dextrose
- lactose (milk sugar)
- molasses
- maple syrup
- corn syrup.

The following are examples of complex carbohydrates:

- wholegrains (e.g. whole wheat, brown rice, oats, barley, rye, corn, millet) and the foods made from them, such as breads and pasta
- beans/legumes
- potatoes.

Simple carbohydrates are forms of sugar which are in a more readily usable form, requiring little effort to metabolize. It is for this reason that they are such an appropriate food source for yeasts. Simple carbohydrates consist of *monosaccharides* (one single sugar molecule) and *disaccharides* (two sugar molecules linked together). In contrast, complex carbohydrates (starches) are comprised of longer chains of sugars containing more molecules. In order to convert carbohydrates into a usable form the digestive system must split them into individual sugar molecules. Naturally, this will be easier and faster to accomplish with a disaccharide than a complex carbohydrate, and fastest with a monosaccharide as it requires no digestion at all.

Sugar Feeds Candida

The main justification for avoiding sugar in your diet is the fact that yeasts such as *Candida albicans* feed on available sugars in your body. The consumption of sugar in even small quantities is enough to promote candidiasis and its debilitating symptoms. In more liberal quantities sugar can, aside from feeding the yeast, weaken your immune and digestive defences against it.

Both you and candida need sugar in order to live; this fact obviously presents a dilemma when you are trying to formulate a candida control diet! Fortunately there is a solution: consume complex rather than simple carbohydrates, as candida cannot efficiently convert complex sugars into a form which they can readily utilize as food.

Another asset to using complex over simple carbohydrates for this purpose stems from their effect on blood sugar. Simple carbohydrates are either broken down quickly or need no breaking down at all, and as such they can be absorbed quickly and provide a nearly immediate and sharp elevation of blood sugar. This is good for the systemic candida but bad for you, and should be avoided at all costs. Complex carbohydrates, on the other hand, are broken down gradually and thus are absorbed and utilized gradually. Ultimately this leads to a more consistent and controlled maintenance of blood sugar – enough to keep your cells functioning with a steady availability of sugar for energy, but not sufficient to encourage a gluttonous population of candida.

Sugar and Gut Fermentation

The fermentation of any form of simple sugar is within the capabilities of *Candida albicans*, leading to the production of alcohol and its toxic by-product, acetaldehyde. The end result of the manufacture of fermentation by-products by candida and certain bacteria are symptoms associated with the condition known as irritable bowel syndrome (IBS) such as diarrhoea and/or constipation, bloating, gas, etc. The bloating, gas, and reflux of stomach acid into the oesophagus are associated with the production of methane, hydrogen and carbon dioxide gases. Alcohol and certain acidic irritants are also produced in the intestines, and may cause gastric spasms leading to diarrhoea or constipation. Intestinal irritants may even promote gut wall damage and excessive permeability. These, added to the toxic 'hangover' effect of acetaldehyde, help to illustrate the negative implications of sugar fermentation in candidiasis.

(For further information you may want to refer to this author's book, *Irritable Bowel Syndrome*.)

Sugar and Immune Function

As if the above concerns were not enough reason to avoid sugar, it can also be devastating to the immune system. This fact has been proven in research which involved observing the effect of sugar on the activity of certain white blood cells (*neutrophils* and *lymphocytes*). As you know, it is the white blood cells that carry out the destruction of invading organisms in the blood; neutrophils and lymphocytes make up the vast majority of all white blood cells in the body.

In the research it was discovered that within half an hour of consuming 100 grams of various types of simple carbohydrates the activity of neutrophils began to drop. At its worst, the level of activity was generally reduced by at least 50 per cent! The immune suppression typically continued for at least five hours. To put this into perspective, 100 g is thought to be only about two-thirds of the average daily intake of miscellaneous sugars. Further study of the effects of smaller amounts of sugar (75-g portions) on lymphocyte activity showed a peak of around 20 per cent reduction. These immuno-suppressive effects occurred with different types of simple carbohydrates such as sucrose, honey, glucose, fructose and even orange juice. It is interesting to note that starch (complex carbohydrate) was tested as well and caused *no* ill-effects on white blood cell activity. As these immune cells are involved in the destruction of systemic candida, anything which inhibits their activity would hamper your recovery, to put it mildly.

Sugar and Adrenal Function

Aside from its nutritional uses as a source of energy, sugar also acts as a stimulant within the body. When sugar is consumed, levels of the hormone *adrenaline* (from the adrenal glands) rise. Adrenaline is the hormone associated with the 'fight or flight' response which occurs in the early stages of a stress reaction. Adrenaline causes the tell-tale symptoms of acute stress such as rapid heartbeat and breathing, sweaty palms, hyper-alertness and extreme tenseness of the nerves and muscles. This may account for at least part of the jitteriness that many people experience if they eat too much sugar at one time.

The effect of adrenaline on muscle and nerve tension may play a key role in exacerbating Irritable Bowel Syndrome. What is less known is the fact that adrenaline also accounts for the shunting of blood away from the digestive system, thus temporarily weakening its function. This is yet another possible negative outcome of consuming large quantities of sugar, at least at any one time. A small amount of sugar is unlikely to have a significant harmful effect on digestion but, as mentioned, even minimal quantities will provide food for the yeast.

There are other concerns regarding excessive sugar ingestion, but the above represent the most important to the control of candidiasis. The bottom line is that if you suffer with candidiasis, then even minimal amounts of sugar should be avoided until reasonable control of the overgrowth has been established. There are stumbling blocks to this important step in your programme, however, and we shall now take a look at some of the most common.

SUGAR CRAVINGS

First of all, the very thought of eliminating sugar is inconceivable to many sufferers, particularly when their candidiasis is systemic. The reason is that systemic candida can cause over-whelming cravings for sugar. This should not be confused with loving sweet-tasting foods or snacks, as people generally find sweet things appealing to the palate. Cravings are different, and the cravings associated with candidiasis can be unbelievably powerful at times.

The significant alterations in endocrine hormones seen in systemic candidiasis can lead to hypoglycaemia (low blood sugar). One of the common symptoms of hypoglycaemia is sugar cravings, presumably in response to the need to elevate the sugar supply in the blood. The problem is that, should you satisfy this craving by eating some sugar, the result is the very vicious circle known as 're-bound hypoglycaemia'. When you eat sugar, blood sugar goes up and the pancreas pumps out the hormone *insulin* in order to facilitate the metabolism of the sugar. Insulin levels can be elevated to such an extent that this causes blood sugar levels to 'crash' again, causing you to crave sugar again, and the cycle continues. Insulin does not influence the sugar in your intestines, working only after it is absorbed into the bloodstream. Naturally this means that the intestinal candida has repeated feasts. Even worse is that if the intestinal candida consumes a great deal of sugar before it is absorbed into your bloodstream, then blood sugar levels will not be elevated commensurate to your sugar intake and your cravings are likely to continue, further strengthening the candida while you get worse and worse.

HIDDEN SUGARS

The commonness of simple carbohydrates makes their elimination very difficult indeed. Even if you previously have made a conscious effort to reduce or eliminate sugar from your diet, sugar (especially sucrose) may be hidden in many prepared foods. A lot of people check labels for sugar; however, some food manufacturers may either inadvertently (or intentionally) give the impression of a 'healthier' product by using the scientific term for a sugar. For example, it is likely that a great many people are unaware that dextrose is a form of sugar. You should also be aware that fructose is sometimes called 'corn sweetener', 'fruit sugar' or *levulose*, and sucrose may be called just 'sugar' on the label of some food products. In the initial stages of your programme, you should shy away from any of these, no matter what they are called!

Please note: If the suffix 'ose' appears at the end of an ingredient this typically signifies a sugar of some sort (such as sucrose, glucose, fructose, lactose, maltose, etc.).

SUGAR SUBSTITUTES

The strong justification against using sugar in any candidiasis control programme will lead many to consider opting for sugar substitutes. The case for or against using them is impossible to assess because each type of substitute has different chemical attributes which will react in the body in different ways, and tolerance to them varies from person to person. The clear advantage that sugar substitutes have over sugar in such a programme is simply the fact that they are not metabolized in the exact same manner as sugar. As a result, they will be treated differently by your body, and by candida. Because of their lack of calorie value (hence their use in diet drinks, etc.), they are unable to supply a significant source of energy, and thus are of little direct use either to you or the candida organism. In spite of this there are certain varieties which should probably be avoided.

Some of the more common sugar substitutes include *sorbitol*, *mannitol*, *xylitol*, *aspartame* and *saccharin*. Sorbitol, mannitol and xylitol are referred to as *sugar alcohols* and are metabolized by the body more like an alcohol than a sugar. They are frequently used in 'sugar free' sweets or chewing gum. Interestingly, it has been shown that sorbitol can produce intestinal distress symptoms in IBS sufferers. Considering this fact, and the chemical nature and metabolism of sugar alcohols, it is probably best to avoid their use when fighting candidiasis.

Aspartame has become the sugar substitute of choice by many food and beverage companies, to a great extent due to its very similar taste to table sugar and low calorie concentration. Aspartame is a chemical comprised of what is known as a *methyl ester* of the amino acids *l-phenylalanine* and *l-aspartic acid*. Aspartame has been the subject of controversy for quite some time due to the growing list of adverse reactions to it. It has been reported that when aspartame is metabolized in the intestines it releases *methanol* (wood alcohol) into the system. It is not the intention of this book to debate its safety; however, especially due to the increased propensity for alcohol sensitivity (see below) and compromised liver function in systemic candidiasis, aspartame is probably best avoided. Saccharin has fallen out of favour over the last several years for various reasons – presumably not least being concern about its safety and the advent of aspartame on the market. Candida will not find it a suitable food source, but as with any sugar substitute if you decide to use it, check your tolerance very closely and use it as infrequently as possible.

Because of the question marks regarding these sugar substitutes, if you can manage without them it would be preferable to do so. In addition, it will probably be much easier to wean yourself away from the 'need' for sweet-tasting foods while your motivation to follow this programme is strongest. Success in adjusting your taste buds will undoubtedly help your efforts to moderate your sugar intake from now on.

How long you should restrict your intake of sugar depends on many factors, especially how successful you are in controlling the proliferation of candida and how well your immune system recovers. Naturally this will vary from person to person – the optimal period of avoidance may be from several weeks to several months. Because there is no 100 per cent accuracy to diagnostic tests, for many the best way of knowing when to reintroduce sugar into the diet is to wait until significant recovery is symptomatically apparent, and then to use trial and error to make any adjustments. The more completely you follow the dietary recommendations in this chapter and the supplemental approach outlined in the next chapter, the sooner you are liable to be able to tolerate sugar.

Whenever you attempt to reinstate sugar into your diet, the process should be slow, gradual and moderate. Should you experience even a small relapse of symptoms after reintroducing sugar in your diet, then eliminate it again immediately for a while until your system is stronger. *It is important to note that, especially after long-term candidiasis, there exists a chance that you will continue to remain at least somewhat sensitive to sugar even after your recovery is complete.*

FRUIT AND FRUIT JUICES

It is clear that sugar presents the main dietary concern, but of course sugar is not restricted to sweeteners. The problem is simple carbohydrates in general, and they are present in fruit and fruit juices as well. The fructose in fruits and fruit juice is fermented by yeast and bacteria, producing the detrimental by-products referred to on many occasions in this book. In some IBS sufferers the improper digestion of the disaccharides fructose or lactose may produce sometimes severe digestive symptoms as well as malabsorption. Experience will tell you whether or not you react adversely to these disaccharides; the difficulty is in knowing whether any adverse symptoms are related to stimulating a feeding frenzy in the yeast colonies or a defect in disaccharide digestion (or both). Either way, eating fruit will feed the candida, and there is strong justification for avoiding fruit and especially fruit juices in the early stages of your programme.

Taking fruit juice or dried fruit is worse than eating a piece of fresh fruit. Fresh fruit contains not only fruit sugar but also dietary fibre and a high percentage of water. These additional attributes serve to dilute the overall concentration of sugar entering your system. Dietary fibre slows the rate at which the food you eat empties from the stomach. This ultimately slows the sugar release to awaiting throngs of hungry yeast in the intestines, as well as slowing the entry of sugar into the bloodstream.

The high water content of fresh fruit also helps to dilute sugar concentration in general. In fruit juice there is water, but little or no fibre; dried fruit contains fibre, but very little water. Dried fruit unfortunately is also a wonderful medium for mould growth. As you would expect, pure fructose (levulose) used as a sweetener is the least desirable as it lacks both water and fibre. Pure fructose also lacks the vitamins and minerals found in fresh fruit.

There are differing opinions among practitioners who treat candidiasis as to whether all fruit should be avoided in the beginning stages of the programme. Some practitioners choose to allow certain fresh fruit (such as apples) in small quantities; however, this does feed the yeast, thus slowing the process of control and recovery to varying degrees, depending on the individual and the type and quantity of fruit consumed. If you decide to choose what seems to be the *optimal* (and fastest) approach, eliminate all fruit and fruit-derived foods for at least the first three to four weeks. When and if you choose to reintroduce it after this time, do it slowly and assess your tolerance. As with sugar, if you experience any sensitivity or even a slight setback, then simply cut it out again and perhaps wait a couple of weeks to a month before attempting it again.

If, however, you find it too overwhelming to avoid fruit altogether, to the extent that you feel inclined to abandon the candida control diet altogether, then allow yourself a little fruit.

Complex Carbohydrates

As you can see, it is not carbohydrates *per se* that are the problem in candidiasis but rather simple carbohydrates, which can be used easily by the yeast as an efficient source of food. Since you require carbohydrates to live, the key is to select a form which is less desirable to the yeast but still able to be used efficiently by your body. The answer is complex carbohydrates (starches). Among the more common and accessible complex carbohydrate sources are:

- cereal grains (such as wheat, rice, oats, barley, rye, corn, millet)
- beans/legumes
- potatoes
- nuts and seeds.

Note that packaged or prepared foods which contain complex carbohydrate sources may also contain sugars. Check labels carefully.

Starch Is Less Attractive to Yeast

The advantage you have over the yeast is your intricate digestive system and all its capabilities. This allows your body to convert more complex foods into simpler forms in a suitable time frame. Once they are broken down, the complex sugars can eventually be utilized by yeast as well, but this is far less conducive to their rapid proliferation and gives your defences what should be ample opportunity to keep the yeast under control.

Blood Sugar Control

As severe fluctuations of blood sugar are one of the main causes of systemic candidiasis symptoms, anything which eradicates this 'rollercoaster ride' of rebound hypoglycaemia will be most welcome to sufferers. There have been many differing philosophies with respect to correcting hypoglycaemia through dietary manipulation, which typically involve adjusting the intake of protein and carbohydrates. In the not too distant past, high protein/ low carbohydrate diets were commonly recommended by dietitians and nutritionists for those with low blood sugar. Since then this approach has been amended by some of the most highly respected nutritional scientists and practitioners to a moderate protein/high *complex* carbohydrate/ *low* simple carbohydrate diet. These experts recognize that the manner in which starches are broken down allows the blood sugar to be elevated gradually, thereby not stimulating the often exceedingly sharp rise in insulin release which accompanies simple carbohydrate intake. This eliminates the 'rebound' effect and all its symptoms. The optimum blood sugar levels can then be maintained for a much longer period of time, without the severe peak which occurs almost immediately after consuming simple sugars. Using complex carbohydrates in this manner may also help moderate your craving for sugar, thus helping you to avoid eating something which you may well regret soon after.

Use 'Wholefood' Starches

All starchy foods are *not* created equal. Well, maybe they are *created* equal, but food manufacturers often change this and concoct a striking difference in some of them – a difference of which you should be aware. In nature, starches are found in foods containing other natural substances which interlink with the starch. These substances, such as fibre, vitamins and minerals, actually affect the manner in which the starch will be digested and metabolized, in your favour. For instance, fibre will further slow the release of the sugars from the food and will even slow the emptying of the food from the stomach into the intestines. Many of the vitamins and minerals in the food play a role in the utilization of the carbohydrates.

Food processing methods often remove these important substances from the 'whole' food, leaving the starch in a form which is converted to simpler sugars more quickly in the digestive tract. Common examples include the conversion of whole wheat into white flour and the creation of white rice from brown rice. As a result, you would be better off favouring, for instance, whole wheat pasta over the processed durum semolina types normally used; and brown rice is far better for you than white rice. Beans and other legumes, and potatoes (in moderation) represent other 'wholefood' starches which can add some versatility to the carbohydrate portion of your diet. Sweet potatoes and yams should be avoided in the earlier stages of the programme, as they contain a fair amount of simpler sugars in addition to starch.

Because the starch molecules will be broken down, albeit slowly, into simpler sugars in the digestive tract, some practitioners who treat candidiasis prefer to moderate their patients' total carbohydrate intake to a maximum of 60–80 g per day in the early stages (that is, the first two to four weeks) of the programme. To put this into perspective, two 50-g servings of brown rice (dry weight) per day would typically supply a total of 70–80 g of carbohydrate. Many, if not most practitioners have excellent success treating candidiasis with no such restriction, provided the intake is in the form of wholefood sources of complex carbohydrates, such as wholegrains, beans/legumes and, occasionally, white potatoes.

ALCOHOL

There are many negative implications of alcohol with respect to candidiasis. Even a minimal amount of alcohol becomes an ever-increasing enemy to the body as candida grows in dominance.

Alcohol Feeds Yeast

Alcohol is a good friend to candida. Beverages such as
beer, wine or spirits provide a form of carbohydrates
which can be readily used by the yeast as a food source.
This reason alone is enough justification to avoid them.
The correlation between sugar, alcohol and yeast is best
illustrated in the use of yeast to ferment carbohydrates in
fruit or malted grains to make various alcoholic beverages.

Alcohol Contains Yeast Constituents

A candidiasis infection will often lead to an allergy to
even non-candida yeasts and yeast constituents. Alcoholic
beverages contain yeast residues and thus may bring
about an adverse reaction irrespective of any part they play
in feeding the candida. Though the yeast may not be
alive at the time of consumption, and thus cannot proliferate, it can still produce a sensitivity reaction. In addition
to the symptoms of the reaction, such allergies will further
drain what may be an already compromised immune
system.

Alcohol and Liver Function

Most people are aware of the fact that drinking alcohol
can have an adverse effect on the liver, but this is usually thought to be associated with excessive alcohol intake.
As it happens, what constitutes 'excessive' alcohol intake
is relative to the individual, and a candidiasis sufferer is
likely to have a much lower tolerance than normal. In this
context, lower tolerance means the reduced ability of
the liver to carry out its intended functions. This said,
those with candidiasis also often become drunk after
comparatively low amounts of alcohol. You may recall the

reported cases of those who became drunk after consuming no alcohol whatsoever.

The liver carries out many functions, but the ones we are most concerned with here are detoxification, and the liver's complementary role in immunity. There are countless toxins you are exposed to on a daily basis: in the environment, in food and water supplies, and those made inside your body during metabolism or by microorganisms. Alcohol metabolism itself provides the liver with one of the most damaging toxins to filter, acetaldehyde. Because alcohol and acetaldehyde are produced anyway as a result of candida overgrowth, this can account for the candidiasis sufferer's extreme sensitivity to even very small amounts of alcohol. When the liver is called upon to carry out the huge task of neutralizing ever-growing amounts of candida-related toxins, it will become less and less efficient at detoxifying poisons or aiding immunity through blood filtration. Interestingly, the link between alcohol and toxicity in the body is not limited to alcohol's effect on liver function, as research shows that the very process of ingesting alcohol causes an increase in the toxins absorbed in the gut.

Alcohol Depletes Nutrients

Alcohol interferes with the metabolism of, and causes the excretion of a wide variety of essential micronutrients (such as vitamins, minerals, fatty acids) which are needed for the maintenance of literally every system and cell of the body. The effect of resulting deficiencies on the digestive, immune and endocrine systems are of particular concern in your recovery. The loss of such nutrients will need to be compensated for. This will be discussed in more depth in the next chapter.

YEAST AND OTHER FUNGI

There are many different types of fungi that we come in contact with one way or another. Some just happen to be in our diet. Aside from the inadvertent contact through the invisible growth of moulds on many of the things we eat, we may also choose to consume members of the fungus family, such as:

- baking yeast (e.g. breads, pastries, etc.)
- yeast used in the production of alcoholic beverages
- nutritional yeast supplements (e.g. brewer's, torula)
- yeast extract (e.g. yeast spreads, miscellaneous food flavourings)
- mushrooms
- mouldy cheese.

It is probably no surprise to learn that foods and products containing these organisms are contraindicated in candidiasis. These foods do not actually feed the candida in the body, but the increased sensitivity candidiasis sufferers are likely to have to the cellular components of various fungi suggests that they are best avoided, at least in the earlier stages of the programme. Later on, when the sufferer is feeling better, then tolerance for non-candida fungi can be more easily assessed, as there will then be less confusion between normal candida symptoms and those caused by any sensitivity to other types of fungi. There is evidence that some people with candidiasis develop intolerance to many different species of fungi (in some, sensitivity to fungi will remain even after the candidiasis is successfully eliminated).

VINEGAR AND OTHER FERMENTED FOODS

Aside from alcohol, other types of fermented foods and beverages can also either promote candida growth and/or contain components which trigger symptoms of a fungal allergy. Vinegar (from apple cider, wine, etc.) is particularly problematic. This means that it is best not only to avoid vinegar, but any foods that contain it, or that have been pickled. Foods or beverages containing malt are also well worth avoiding as they provide carbohydrates in a form which is easily converted to food by yeast. Other examples of fermented foods or those containing fermented ingredients include several condiments (ketchup, mustard, relish), many salad dressings, sauerkraut, soy sauce, miso (fermented soybean paste) and amazake (from fermented rice).

DAIRY PRODUCTS

Although not as important as the restriction of simple carbohydrates or alcohol, the elimination of most dairy products would be recommended for an effective anti-candida programme. For one thing, milk and milk-containing foods are the most common cause of food sensitivities – some which are allergic and others which are metabolic in nature.

Lactose and Casein

Milk contains the disaccharide *lactose*, which would best be avoided due to its ability to provide a food source for yeast within the gut. Lactose is also responsible for the most common cause of milk intolerance, whereby the body cannot split the disaccharide into its individual sugar molecules. Lactose intolerance, which is not allergic in nature, leads to symptoms such as gas, abdominal bloating and diarrhoea. *Casein*, the most prominent protein in milk, is typically the cause of allergic milk reactions. Damage to the intestinal mucosa, such as that seen in long-term candidiasis, can inhibit the activity of enzymes which digest disaccharides as well as increasing the absorption of allergy-causing proteins. It is also important to note that dairy cheeses are highly susceptible to mould. All of these concerns suggest that dairy products may well be problematic, at least in the earlier stages of an anti-candida programme.

'Live' Yoghurt

One possible exception to the general restriction of dairy products is live yoghurt. 'Live' refers to the presence of active bacterial cultures in the yoghurt. The bacteria used in yoghurt production are usually related to the beneficial lactobacillus colonies in your digestive tract. As you know, these friendly bacteria play a major role in preventing the overgrowth of *Candida albicans*. The lactobacilli in yoghurt also help digest milk sugar by producing the enzyme *lactase*, which splits the lactose. In spite of its simple carbohydrate content, on balance live yoghurt would be suitable in an anti-candida programme. However, if you are allergic to casein in milk, dairy yoghurt should be avoided as the bacteria will not offset the allergy. Finding yoghurt is easy; finding yoghurt which has live cultures at the time of purchase is not so simple. Check the label closely for this distinction. Your local health food store is likely to have a selection of live yoghurt products. Make certain to select the plain, unsweetened variety. If you happen to be allergic to milk, unsweetened, non-dairy yoghurt made from soybeans is available at many health food stores.

MEAT, POULTRY, ETC.

The growing movement in Western society towards reducing the intake of red meat should be seen as a positive step toward better health. In the case of candidiasis, there are both advantages and disadvantages to cutting meat out of the diet. On the one hand, the regular consumption of red meat does little to maintain the optimal health and function of the digestive tract. On the other hand, meat does not provide food for the candida. The restrictive nature of the candida control diet obviously makes it more difficult to create a meal plan which is practical, appealing and, above all, does not feed the yeast in your gut.

Red meat is difficult to digest and is especially difficult to eliminate from the intestinal tract. Because of this, it can be antagonistic to the health of the digestive tract, especially for a person who already has the disadvantage of a yeast overgrowth. As a result, it would be preferable to opt for other forms of concentrated protein such as fish and poultry, which will be easier on the system and also will not feed the yeast. You do not necessarily have to eliminate red meat from your diet completely, but try to restrict yourself to two or three times a week. There are plenty of alternative sources of dietary protein, such as poultry, fish, eggs (not raw), beans/legumes, and nuts and seeds (freshly shelled). When selecting from this list, there are a few important tips to be aware of.

1 When selecting meat or poultry it is recommended that you find a source which has not been treated with drugs. It is common practice in commercial rearing of cattle and chickens to use antibiotics to control disease and certain hormones to stimulate growth. As a result, it would be better to find meat or poultry

that is untreated if possible (that is, organic).

2 Eggs are a very good source of protein, but under no circumstances are they to be eaten raw. Raw egg whites contain a substance called *avidin* which blocks the utilization of *biotin*, a B vitamin that is essential in preventing the conversion of simple candida cells into the mycelial fungal form (*see Chapter 9*). Biotin is also necessary for proper protein utilization.

3 If you are using members of the bean/legume family as a major source of protein, make sure you are getting ample levels of 'complete' protein – that is, adequate levels of all eight essential amino acids. In general, combining a bean/legume with a wholegrain (such as kidney beans and brown rice) will give you a complete protein; however, soybeans can stand alone as a complete protein source.

4 When nuts and seeds have been liberated from their shells, they soon become a suitable medium for the growth of moulds. As a result, any nuts and seeds should be eaten at the time of shelling. Peanuts and pistachios, which are especially susceptible to significant mould levels, should probably be avoided completely.

VEGETABLES

Most vegetables can be consumed liberally, especially those of the green, leafy variety such as broccoli, spinach, kale, leaf lettuce, endive, miscellaneous greens, watercress, parsley, etc. Cauliflower, cabbage and cucumber are also excellent. Onions and many spices (such as garlic, ginger and rosemary) can be eaten freely, especially for their inhibiting effect on pathogenic organisms (*see Chapter 9 for a discussion of garlic*).

In general, vegetables are rich in vitamins, minerals

and fibre, and they often contain very powerful antioxidant substances which help counteract the negative effects of free radicals in the body. Most of them will not feed the yeast. If you experience extreme chemical sensitivity, it would be best to use organic vegetables whenever possible. If organic produce is unavailable to you, scrub any commercial vegetables very thoroughly to remove as many surface pesticides or chemical fertilizers as possible (be aware that some chemicals can permeate vegetables and fruit, and thus will not be removed by scrubbing).

FATTY FOODS

Because the activity of the digestive tract is so essential to the control of candida overgrowth, it is best to avoid anything that impairs this process. The excessive consumption of fatty foods is a case in point. In a heavily fatty meal, the fat slows down the digestion of the other foods eaten and can produce irregular intestinal contractions as well. This does not mean, however, that you should avoid fat altogether; only that you should eat it in moderation.

It has been observed in research that many candidiasis sufferers have a deficiency in the *omega-3* class of fatty acids. These individuals have also been shown to display excessive levels of *arachidonic acid*, a fatty acid of the *omega-6* variety. Such abnormalities are thought to be due to metabolic factors related to the candidiasis. Arachidonic acid (AA) is an unsaturated fatty acid which is made in small quantities in your body through the metabolism of other *omega-6* fatty acids in your diet. The quantity of AA to be made is limited by certain metabolic controls. However, arachidonic acid is also prevalent in animal fats. As a result you should restrict the amount of animal fats you eat, so that levels of AA are not too high in your system. Reducing your intake of red meat and dairy products would help in lowering AA levels. The white meat of poultry is preferable because of its lower total fat percentage compared to that of dark poultry meat. Fish would be better still and, as it happens, certain types of fish (such as salmon, mackerel, herring, tuna, cod, etc.) are excellent sources of the *omega-3* fatty acids which, as mentioned, appear to be deficient in many candidiasis sufferers. The consumption of fried or excessively heated unsaturated fats should be reduced, as this damages the beneficial attributes the fats may have had prior to cooking and actually makes them unhealthy to the body in many ways.

Many practitioners suggest taking raw, unrefined virgin olive oil as an aid to candidiasis treatment. Oleic acid, a prominent fatty acid in olive oil, has been reported to help prevent the conversion of the simple candida cell into its mycelial fungal form.

TEA AND COFFEE

Tea and coffee may not be sweet, but they are a suitable medium for mould growth. Actually, the standard types of black tea are themselves fermented. Black tea starts off as green tea, which is then fermented to produce the distinctive flavour and colour of black tea. Its caffeine content may also be problematic for some sufferers, in part because caffeine acts as an adrenal stimulant and, as such, may exacerbate the stress-linked symptoms of candidiasis. In liberal quantities, caffeine may also trigger blood sugar fluctuations as it causes stored sugar to be dumped out of the liver into the bloodstream. This, in turn, brings about insulin release and can result in a drop in blood sugar. Small amounts of caffeine are unlikely to create much of a problem for the average person, but those with candidiasis are likely to be more sensitive to it. Another concern is that tea and coffee inhibit the absorption of the trace mineral *zinc* – which is, among other things, necessary for proper immune and digestive function.

If you want to drink tea, then consider one of the caffeine-free herbal varieties (though not those derived from fruits). If you still want some caffeine in spite of any potential harm it can do, then green tea would be a better option as it is not fermented and possesses certain health benefits. If you drink a great deal of coffee and find it hard to eliminate it completely from your diet, you may prefer to wean yourself off it gradually. If you do so, the fresher the coffee, the less susceptible it is to mould. Try to buy the freshest whole beans and grind them yourself each time you want a cup. It would still be best, however to eliminate coffee completely as soon as you can.

SMOKING

Aside from the well-documented risks of lung cancer, emphysema, cardiovascular disease, etc. smoking can also present significant problems to the candidiasis sufferer. Among other things, smoking drains several essential nutrients from the body that are needed for the proper function of the immune and digestive systems. These systems can also be adversely affected by the inadvertent release of adrenal hormones in response to nicotine.

Damaging molecules or molecular fragments known as free radicals in cigarette smoke inhibit the repair of connective tissue, which is also compromised by the loss of vitamin C caused by smoking (vitamin C is needed to make collagen, the main protein in connective tissue). This directly affects the lungs and the entire respiratory tract, and would indirectly influence the health of connective tissue in other parts of the body, such as the intestinal wall. Systemic candidiasis often leads to respiratory symptoms anyway (such as sinusitis, catarrh) even in those who do not smoke. Aside from free radicals, cigarette smoke contains many noxious chemicals and heavy metals. These may, at least in part, account for the common complaint of extreme sensitivity to cigarette smoke in non-smoking candidiasis sufferers.

FOLLOWING THE DIET

Once you begin your own candidiasis programme it is important to follow the restrictions listed here as consistently as possible until you have gained adequate control over the intestinal overgrowth – and if it is systemic, until your immune system and other bodily processes have recovered adequately. The length of time it takes before the body can tolerate restricted foods varies greatly from person to person, so there is no way to recommend a standard period of time that applies to all sufferers. Nevertheless, it is often suggested that a strict adherence to the diet is advisable for at least the first three months. The more severe the case (that is, systemic candidiasis), the longer the restrictions should be adhered to for the best results. The avoidance of yeast-feeding foods is the most important dietary feature of any anti-candida regime. It is important to note that even long after the body has recovered, you may still remain sensitive to certain foods. Trial and error may be the easiest way to refine your diet after the main restrictions are lifted, but if many sensitivities persist it may be a good idea to embark on food sensitivity testing. (For more information on food allergy and intolerance testing, you may want to refer to this author's book, *Allergies*.)

For the optimal results it is best to consume any food soon after you prepare it, as moulds can grow quickly on 'leftovers'. Drink plenty of water (at least six to eight glasses per day), but preferably not during meals as this can dilute stomach acidity (needed for digesting your food). It is recommended you drink purified or bottled (preferably non-carbonated) water. The chemicals used in treating tap water may not be well tolerated by some who are chemically sensitive, and chlorine (used to kill water-borne bacteria) is unlikely to do your digestive bacteria any good either.

The choice of just how strictly you follow the programme is up to you, and only you. 'Cheating' in the early stages of your programme, especially with sugar, can set you back considerably in your progress; however, if you do happen to falter, forget about it and just start back on your programme as though nothing has happened. It is very, very counterproductive to your efforts to feel guilty, hopeless or as though you have ruined everything. Such psychological self-torture is unlikely to motivate you to get back on track; it is more likely to make you give up completely. Remember, the fact that you are reading this book in the first place shows that you have chosen to take control and responsibility for your health and well-being. This is something to be proud of, especially as it is the first, and often the most difficult step towards recovery.

CHAPTER 9

Nutritional and Herbal Therapies

Ever since C. Orian Truss M.D. published his ground-breaking book *The Missing Diagnosis* in 1982, more and more medical doctors and natural medicine practitioners have become cognizant of the scope of candidiasis. *The Yeast Connection* by William Crook M.D. (1983) followed on from Dr Truss' work to help many understand this condition better. It is not that *Candida albicans* or even candidiasis was a new discovery at the time; research into the treatment of candida infections had already been published decades before. What Truss and Crook *did* uncover was the nearly unlimited range of such infections and the fact that yeast overgrowth can cause a previously unrecognized syndrome involving many different symptoms and body systems. In their books they describe the condition and several case histories to highlight their observations; they also discuss prospective treatment programmes and their clinical efficacy. The updated version of *The Yeast Connection* (1986; see also Crook's *The Yeast Connection and the Woman*, 1995) is especially interesting in this respect, in that Dr Crook has included feedback from readers of earlier editions of the book, as well as interviews he has conducted with many other experts in the field on the success of various treatments.

NYSTATIN AND NIZORAL

As Truss and Crook are both orthodox medical doctors, their works focus a great deal of attention on the employment of prescription anti-fungal drugs such as *nystatin* and *nizoral*. They also discuss the necessity of avoiding certain foods and even the potential value of certain natural therapies involving nutritional and/or herbal supplementation. It is important to be aware of nystatin and nizoral as they are still the treatments of choice of many orthodox medical practitioners, even some of those who are orientated more towards natural medicine.

Nystatin is a drug which kills yeast on direct contact. When it is administered internally it is absorbed very poorly in the intestines. One disadvantage of this poor absorption is that, unless very large amounts are used, there will be minimal affect on systemic candida or on those organisms which succeed in penetrating deeper into the intestinal mucosa. There are some who suggest that nystatin may in fact force more candida deeper into the tissues. The advantage of the poor absorption of this drug is that, because less enters the blood, there is more nystatin to saturate the intestines. At any rate, nystatin is effective at clearing surface candida cells. Although nystatin appears to be one of the safer drugs of this nature, high doses can cause side-effects such as nausea in some people.

Nizoral is also effective at killing yeast. Its advantage over nystatin is that it is much better absorbed in the intestines, thus being more effective at dealing with both deeply embedded and systemic candida. On the other hand, nizoral is more likely to produce side-effects due to toxins produced from the 'die off' of candida (Herxheimer reaction).

In spite of the effectiveness of nystatin and nizoral,

they do have their limitations and liabilities. They are generally safer and are tolerated better than many other prescription drugs, but they are not free of side-effects or toxicity; it has also been suggested that stopping long-term nystatin treatment may lead to candida re-establishing itself more strongly than before treatment.

NATURAL THERAPIES

Fortunately, published research has uncovered many natural substances which also possess anti-fungal properties; some are nutritional, some are plant-derived and still others are made in the body, and all can be taken in a supplemental form to comprise a safe and effective anti-candida programme. Unlike nystatin and nizoral, certain nutritional and herbal substances are known to strengthen the immune system directly, help repair damaged tissues, improve digestion, etc. regardless of their effect on candida, and generally support the body in a manner that aids in the recovery from candidiasis.

The nutrients, herbs and other natural substances discussed below are considered to be very safe and do not involve a high risk of side-effects or toxicity.

Probiotics

It is clear that adverse changes in the 'balance of power' in the intestinal tract are standard features in candidiasis. There are many factors which may swing the balance in favour of the candida, such as the use of prescribed antibiotics. Whatever the cause of the imbalance, it is vital that this problem be addressed in order to treat the infection successfully. Killing the yeast (whether with drugs or natural alternatives) is part of the process, but it is also necessary to repopulate the intestinal tract with the friendly types of organisms which, in a healthy person, function to control the yeast. It is one thing to kill the yeast, but you will not obliterate it permanently from your body. As a result, if you do not reinstate the bacterial defence system which human beings normally possess, any residual candida will take over once again. In addition, beneficial bacteria play many other important roles in our health, and are therefore useful over and above their role in fighting candida.

Supplements which put the beneficial bacteria back into your intestines are often referred to as *probiotics*. Probiotics may comprise one or sometimes many different types of bacteria, each with its own unique beneficial functions within the intestines (beneficial bacteria may function in other areas as well, such as the vaginal canal). In the case of candidiasis, the two most important classes of bacteria used in probiotic supplements include:

lactobacillus species – especially *Lactobacillus acidophilus* and *Lactobacillus bulgaricus*
bifidobacterium species – such as *Bifidobacterium bifidum* and *Bifidobacterium longum*.

The disruption of the population of beneficial bacteria does more than just encourage the overgrowth of *Candida albicans* and its damaging effects. It also creates a more suitable environment for the overgrowth of other pathogenic organisms such as harmful bacteria and intestinal worms and protozoa. Candida and the other pathogenic species have anything but a symbiotic relationship with your body – they are parasites, pure and simple, and they will flourish only at the expense of your health.

The problems caused by pathogenic bacteria further encourage the difficulties caused by candida, both in the intestines and systemically. For example, the production of polyamines (from the bacterial breakdown of protein components) can encourage excessive intestinal permeability, and when systemic is associated with triggering the skin disorder psoriasis as well as certain forms of arthritis.

Friendly bacteria maintain a less pathogenic environment in the gut. There are a few different ways which they accomplish this task with respect to *Candida albicans*, and we shall take a look at three of these ways now.

1 COMPETITION FOR FOOD

As you know, sugars are the preferred food of *Candida albicans*. Beneficial bacteria also thrive on available sugars in the gut. As a result, these organisms must compete for available food. The greater the numbers of beneficial bacteria in the gut, the less food there will be for candida to thrive on. The converse is true as well, so one of the keys to treatment is stacking the numbers in favour of the 'good guys'. This 'numbers game' is even more important when you consider that the friendly organisms are competing not only with candida but with other pathogenic organisms.

2 COMPETITION FOR SPACE

Organisms such as candida also need a place to live in order to establish themselves in the intestinal environment. They take up residence on the surface of intestinal mucosa in a process known as implantation. It is from this implantation site that they can eventually penetrate through the gut walls in their mycelial form. Without an opportunity to implant, they cannot remain in the intestines to feed and proliferate, and are then easier to eliminate through the stool. The two main beneficial strains of bacteria in the small and large intestines (*Lactobacillus acidophilus* and *bifidobacteria* respectively) also implant, and in adequate numbers can thus lessen the implantation capabilities of candida.

3 CREATING AN UNDESIRABLE ENVIRONMENT FOR CANDIDA

Certain types of friendly bacteria discourage populations not only of yeast but of other harmful organisms by making the environment of the intestines inhospitable. Restricting food supply and implantation space are not the only methods; another method is by altering the pH (acid-alkaline balance) of the intestinal tract. Candida thrives better in a higher pH (more alkaline); friendly bacteria can produce substances such as *lactic acid* which lower the intestinal pH and drive out candida in the process. Some beneficial organisms also produce natural antibiotic substances which help control pathogenic bacteria.

Aside from killing yeast directly, the key to creating a balance in favour of the friendly bacteria is to ingest them as a concentrated supplement. Such supplementation should preferably include the types of bacteria discussed below.

Lactobacillus Acidophilus

Lactobacillus acidophilus is the major beneficial bacteria in the small intestine. It is both an acid-loving and lactic acid-producing bacteria, and as such helps create an upper intestinal pH which is not conducive to candida survival. *L. acidophilus* also competes for food and uses up valuable implantation space in the approximately 20-ft (7-m) long small intestine. As the small intestine is the site of most digestion and absorption of food nutrients, and makes up the vast majority of the digestive tract, protection of this environment is especially important to your overall state of health.

Certain strains of *L. acidophilus* also produce chemicals which kill pathogenic bacteria. Additionally, *L. acidophilus* manufactures the enzyme lactase, and as such can benefit those with lactose intolerance.

Bifidobacteria

Bacteria abound in the large intestine, and it is here that the family of microflora known as bifidobacteria (*Bifidobacterium bifidum* and *Bifidobacterium longum*) help create a healthy environment amid stiff competition. Like *L. acidophilus*, bifidobacteria compete with candida for food and implantation space, and lower the pH of the large intestine to an acidity which is unfavourable to candida. Bifidobacteria (bifidum and certain other forms) are by far the dominant organisms in the large intestines of babies who are breast-fed. This is thought to afford breast-fed babies a greater resistance to infections. Bifidobacteria remain the primary protective force in the colon of healthy adults; however, it appears that the numbers of bifidobacteria are prone to drop off markedly as we get older.

Lactobacillus Bulgaricus

Lactobacillus bulgaricus is a type of bacteria often used in the culturing of yoghurt products. Unlike *L. acidophilus* it does not implant, but rather functions as a transient bacteria, meaning it carries out its functions (such as carbohydrate digestion) while travelling through the intestinal tract without attaching to any specific site. As a lactic bacteria,

L. bulgaricus can help produce an intestinal pH unfavourable to various pathogenic species, and will also take part in the competition for food.

CHOOSING PROBIOTIC SUPPLEMENTATION

Research has shown that concentrated dry cultures of viable probiotics are effective in inhibiting the growth and survival of *Candida albicans*. These results occurred both *in vitro* (tests performed outside the body) as well as in human studies, and demonstrated that successful inhibition of candida could be achieved either by ingestion or local administration (such as vaginal implantation for a local yeast infection).

Although live yoghurt will provide some of these organisms, and has been used successfully in some studies, when using probiotics therapeutically supplementation with concentrated dry cultures would seem preferable. For one thing, dry cultures often provide viable organisms in much higher potencies than are found in yoghurt products. Also, it is easier to determine accurately the potency of a dry culture. Additionally, a wider selection of different organisms is available in powdered form (whether encapsulated or non-encapsulated).

The most important criteria in a probiotic product is that the organisms in the product are live. Being aware of a few other important parameters will help you to select the most suitable probiotic product for your needs. For example, you will want to address the environment in both the small and large intestines. Because of the popularity of *L. acidophilus* (typically called just 'acidophilus'), often bifidobacteria are neglected in supplementation. Considering the fact that the large intestine (where bifidobacteria function) is typically the original site from which candida proliferates, it is well worth ensuring its proper bacterial balance. Though most studies focus on *L. acidophilus*, research does confirm that bifidobacteria successfully control candida as well. Even using one or the other family should help, but it is likely that the best results will be achieved with a combined approach.

In spite of the fact that these beneficial bacteria create an environment which is too acidic for candida, they are normally themselves sensitive to extreme acidity, such as that which is produced in the stomach in order to digest proteins. Because of this, in order to achieve the best results it is important to use bacterial strains which have been tested and shown to possess adequate resistance to the digestive process. Acidophilus and bifidobacteria also need to implant, so you will want to look for probiotics which have been tested to ensure that they successfully implant in the digestive tract.

Probiotic supplements are often cultured on milk, and although this may not present a problem to many candidiasis sufferers, to be on the safe side it may be preferable to choose one of the supplements on the market which is cultured on a milk-free medium (such products typically specify 'non-dairy' or 'milk-free' on the label).

Caprylic Acid

Caprylic acid is a fatty acid found naturally in certain tropical oils such as coconut and palm. It has been used for many years by orthodox doctors and natural medicine practitioners in the treatment of candidiasis. Its therapeutic value in candidiasis is backed by research showing that caprylic acid possesses significant anti-fungal properties.

EARLY RESEARCH

Such research is not at all new, as studies published almost 50 years ago found caprylic acid to be efficacious in treating candida infections. One study published in *The Bulletin of Johns Hopkins Hospital* in 1946 showed considerable benefits in treating active and advancing candida infection, even in cases which were previously unresponsive to standard treatments. Research published in 1954 in the medical journal *Archives of Internal Medicine* also reported the dramatic benefits of this natural therapy. This study, involving patients being treated for substantial intestinal candida overgrowth, reported a total disappearance of *Candida albicans* in stool cultures after patients were treated with caprylic acid.

CAPRYLIC ACID AS A SUPPLEMENT

Today, caprylic acid has established itself as one of the natural treatments of choice in candidiasis therapy. The fact that it is available without a prescription allows many sufferers to have an easily accessible anti-fungal alternative to drugs such as nystatin. Fortunately it appears to be very safe, and is generally well tolerated. Minor side-effects, such as digestive irritation and temporary 'die off' symptoms (often lasting a few days to a week) have been reported in some people, but there appear to be no major health concerns connected with caprylic acid.

Being a fatty acid, caprylic acid is absorbed in the small intestine. Because you want it to reach the large intestine in order to work on the candida colonies thriving there, it is very important to use a caprylic acid supplement which has been specially manufactured to allow adequate caprylic acid to reach the large intestine (this will often be designated on the label).

Aside from caprylic acid, nature has also given us many herbal substances which kill yeast and other pathogenic organisms. Used properly, the benefits of such natural agents can be great, and many of them possess powerful immune-stimulating effects as well.

Goldenseal

One of the most powerful and versatile of all medicinal herbs is goldenseal root (*hydrastis canadensis*). Its uses in traditional herbalism have been wide ranging, and fortunately a great deal of scientific research has confirmed that the active constituents of goldenseal possess a great many medicinal properties, including several relevant to the treatment of candidiasis.

ANTI-MICROBIAL EFFECTS

The main active constituents in goldenseal are the alkaloids *berberine*, *canadine* and *hydrastine*. Berberine, in particular, has been the subject of a huge body of research and has been found to possess a very powerful anti-microbial action. Berberine is the epitome of a full-spectrum anti-microbial in that it can effectively kill many types of yeasts and other fungi (including *Candida albicans*), harmful bacteria, viruses and other parasitic organisms. It appears that berberine's antibacterial effects do not harm beneficial bacteria. Berberine has also been shown to be effective in ameliorating diarrhoea when due to various pathogenic organisms that lead to intestinal infections.

IMMUNE SUPPORT

The ability of berberine to kill candida on contact is further augmented systemically by virtue of the fact that goldenseal also is a powerful stimulant of the immune system. Goldenseal alkaloids have been shown to increase the activity of white blood cells such as macrophages, which devour invading organisms such as candida. The berberine alkaloid also accounts for increased activity of the spleen, where many foreign invaders are disposed of through the action of white blood cells. It also encourages the release of various potent immune substances from the spleen. The antibiotic and immune-stimulating properties of goldenseal make it a popular therapy for infections; using it should make yeast-promoting, broad-spectrum antibiotic drugs unnecessary in many cases (especially in minor infections).

GOLDENSEAL AND LIVER FUNCTION

The anti-fungal effects of goldenseal make it a very attractive option in any anti-candida programme; however, ordinarily the strong candida-killing agents would be inclined to induce the temporary 'die-off' effects of the toxins being released by the dying yeast. Fortunately, goldenseal may be far less prone to causing such symptoms due to the ability of berberine to encourage liver detoxification. The liver is responsible for eliminating die-off toxins from the blood (such toxins are either absorbed from the intestines or produced directly in the blood). Goldenseal is also known to inhibit the production of polyamines, thereby helping to spare the liver (and the intestinal tissue) from yet another challenge. Also relevant is the ability of goldenseal to stimulate bile activity. Bile, a substance made in the liver, helps in the metabolism of dietary fat. Bile is also important to candida control, as it helps deter candida growth in the small intestine. As the liver of a candidiasis sufferer is under constant strain, the additional fortification from goldenseal's active components is especially helpful.

Goldenseal can be used both internally (as capsules or tea) and externally (as a vaginal douche or mouthwash). When taken internally, most people prefer a capsule form due to the incredibly bitter taste of the herb. If used regularly in high doses, it would be advisable to increase your intake of B vitamins, as high levels of berberine are thought to be able to interfere with the body's ability to use B vitamins effectively. The internal use of goldenseal is contraindicated if you are pregnant.

If you use this herb as a vaginal douche or mouthwash the strengths may vary, but you may consider the following approach: Boil one pint (300 ml) of pure water. Take the water off the heat and immediately add the powdered goldenseal (2,000–4,000 mg/2–4 g may be appropriate) and let it steep until the water turns cool. Strain this 'tea' through a coffee filter. Apply once or twice per day (note that if spilled it will stain light-coloured clothing).

Pau d'Arco

South America has provided herbal medicine with many promising discoveries over the years. A Brazilian tree bark, *pau d'arco* (*tabebuia avellendae* or *heptaphylla*) is one such example which pertains to candidiasis. This herb, also known as lapacho or taheebo, has gained notoriety over the last several years based to a great extent on its potential applications in cancer therapy. Research has demonstrated that active constituents of pau d'arco, such as lapachol, naphthoquinones and xyloidine, destroy *Candida albicans*, helping to justify the extensive use of pau d'arco in the natural treatment of candidiasis.

In order to achieve a higher concentration of active

constituents from the herb, pau d'arco is very often decoct-
ed as a strong tea for medicinal purposes; for the sake of
convenience, many prefer to use dried and encapsulated
extracts of pau d'arco. If you prefer to make the tea, the
pau d'arco typically comes as shavings of the bark which
must be simmered in pure water for a minimum of five
minutes. The taste of pau d'arco may take some getting
used to, so if you prefer a weaker tea you may want to
simmer about 10 g of bark in about 16 fl oz (500 ml) of
water for five minutes. For a stronger tea, many prefer to
use up to 20 g of bark, simmered in the same amount of
water for 10–15 minutes. This tea can also be used externally (as a vaginal douche or mouthwash) if desired.

Echinacea

The herb echinacea (*E. purpurea, E. angustifolia*) possesses
an impressive array of immune-stimulating properties.
Many studies have shown that echinacea:

- stimulates white blood cell production and activity
- stimulates the production of interferon
- increases the migration of white blood cells to areas of
  infection
- improves antibody binding
- demonstrates various other properties relevant to
  immune function.

Such a generalized boosting of immune potential would
make echinacea appropriate for aiding in the removal
of systemic candida. As a matter of fact, experimental research suggests that echinacea increases the activity of
phagocytes against *Candida albicans*. Phagocytes are a class
of white blood cells which literally engulf foreign matter in
the lymphatic system.

It is apparently quite common for certain herpes-class viruses associated with ME (chronic fatigue syndrome) to proliferate side by side with systemic candidiasis. Which infection comes first depends on the person, but in any case a top priority would be to enhance the ability of the immune system to attack quickly and destroy efficiently the invading organisms. Research bears out echinacea's safety, and suggests that it would be highly beneficial in the fight against both candidiasis and ME.

Garlic

Not only is garlic one of the most popular spices for cooking, it also happens to possess some of the most significant health benefits of any common herb. Its scientifically-proven attributes are wide reaching, with some of the most heavily researched including protection against cardiovascular disease and broad-spectrum anti-microbial activity.

Garlic's many benefits to health are attributed to various sulphur-based active constituents, which also account for the well-recognized smell of this herb. It has been confirmed that certain garlic components can kill many types of harmful bacteria, viruses, parasitic worms, protozoa and fungi. As a matter of fact, it has been suggested in research that garlic may possess an anti-candida activity stronger than that of nystatin. In addition to garlic supplements, it may be helpful to add generous amounts of freshly minced garlic to your diet.

Milk Thistle

As you know, supporting the detoxification processes of the liver is a special priority in candidiasis. Whether during the worst stages of infection or the die-off stages after treatment starts, candida-related toxins pose a significant challenge to the liver. The active constituents of the herb *milk thistle* (collectively known as *silymarin*) have been proven to possess remarkable liver-protective effects.

One of the most important detoxification substances manufactured in the body is *glutathione*. It has been shown that taking silymarin can increase glutathione levels in the liver by more than 35 per cent. Glutathione is not only involved in detoxification, but also serves as a potent inhibitor of free radical damage (see **Antioxidants**, below). Quite remarkably, silymarin has also been found to stimulate the manufacture of new, healthy liver cells to replace damaged ones. This facility is especially important in cases where the liver may have been significantly compromised due to an especially long-standing candidiasis infection. As silymarin stimulates improved bile flow, it provides additional protection against candida overgrowth in the small intestine.

Silymarin has been used clinically for treating various liver disorders such as hepatitis, cirrhosis and alcoholic liver damage. Its role in enhancing the levels of glutathione in the body and, as a result, increase the liver's ability to eliminate toxins, justifies its use in helping to alleviate chemical sensitivities (common in candidiasis) and 'die-off' effects from candidiasis treatment.

There are many other herbs which possess anti-candida effects or support immune, digestive or detoxification processes, but the above represent some of the most heavily researched, safest and most versatile for internal and/or external use. Aside from the natural agents mentioned above, there are many nutritional agents which should be employed for the most successful anti-candida programme.

Dietary Fibre

Dietary fibre is the primarily indigestible portion of non-animal foods such as wholegrains, vegetables, fruit, beans/legumes and nuts and seeds. It is important to stress *whole* grains here, as the fibre is often removed in various food-processing methods, such as in the conversion of whole wheat into white flour or brown rice into white rice. Fibre serves a multitude of beneficial functions in the human body, which vary somewhat depending on the form of dietary fibre you consume.

INSOLUBLE FIBRE

Insoluble fibre is one of the two major classes of dietary fibre. Cellulose, which is the most common form of insoluble fibre, is a component of plant cell walls. Insoluble fibre is, for the most part, not soluble in water and maintains its consistency throughout the digestive tract.

The main function of insoluble fibre is to facilitate and speed the passage of food through the digestive tract. As it moves through the intestines it takes with it a great deal of water and adds weight to the stool. This is primarily why it helps alleviate constipation, although cellulose (such as from wheat bran) may exacerbate diarrhoea. Insoluble fibre can help cleanse the intestinal walls of waste material and harmful organisms. It can also promote health by aiding in the production of important short-chain fatty acids. Insoluble fibre possesses an impressive list of benefits, but there are times when it is inappropriate in concentrated amounts – and some people find large amounts to be irritating. As it happens, there is another form of fibre which is considerably more suitable to an anti-candidiasis programme. This other form is known as soluble fibre.

SOLUBLE FIBRE

This form of fibre is rich in beans/legumes, certain fruit and vegetables, seeds, and some cereals (especially oats). The physical consistency of soluble fibre is quite different to that of the insoluble form. When soluble fibre is exposed to water it absorbs the moisture and swells in volume, and develops a soft, gel-like texture.

Soluble fibre promotes the fast and easy movement of food through the digestive tract, without irritation, and helps to remove waste material, harmful organisms, etc. Additionally, the resulting increase in stool weight and moisture content helps prevent constipation. Unlike the insoluble form, soluble fibre's sponge-like characteristics and soothing texture help to form the stool properly and reduce diarrhoea. This ability to treat both constipation *and* diarrhoea make soluble fibre especially appropriate for candidiasis sufferers, who often experience both problems alternately (this is a classic feature of Irritable Bowel Syndrome). Because of the significant absorptive properties of soluble fibre, it can be very helpful in binding certain toxins produced in the intestinal tract before they get absorbed into the bloodstream. Considering that toxins which can produce die-off symptoms may originate in the intestines, soluble fibre may help to substantially reduce the severity of such symptoms. In addition, it may help to reduce the irritation associated with intestinally-produced by-products of candida and of the bacterial fermentation of sugars (such as harsh acids, alcohol, gases, etc.). Soluble fibre has even been shown to help regulate blood sugar levels.

Psyllium seed husks represent one of the best supplemental sources of both soluble and insoluble fibre. Psyllium is readily available in the form of either powder or capsules. If you use the powder, it must be mixed with liquid and drunk immediately. If you wait too long to drink it, it will quickly gel, and you will find yourself eating it instead! In the first stages of your programme it is best to mix the powder in pure water rather than fruit juice. Alternatively, you may prefer to avoid its texture and taste (which is not offensive, but not enjoyable either) and use psyllium husk capsules. Regardless of which form you use, it is important to drink a full glass of water after taking the psyllium, in order to achieve the best results.

Digestive Enzymes

The role of digestive secretions in controlling the spread of *Candida albicans* is one of the most important factors to address when looking at both the cause and the treatment of candidiasis. As mentioned in Chapter 5 there are various antagonists to digestive strength, such as stress, antacids, nutrient deficiencies and improper dietary management. Aside from candida overgrowth itself, some of the other common consequences of deficiencies in digestive enzymes include chronic indigestion, gas or bloating soon after eating; chronic constipation and/or diarrhoea; malabsorption; and a tendency to have food allergies.

As a result of the fact that candida can also proliferate in the small intestine and the stomach when digestion is weak, there is a need to focus on reinstating proper digestive activity. Aside from removing obstacles which harm digestion (such as nutrient deficiencies and a poor diet), supplemental replacement of digestive enzymes may yield great benefits in both controlling candida overgrowth and reducing digestive symptoms.

HYDROCHLORIC ACID

Hydrochloric acid (HCL) represents the main digestive and candida-controlling acid in the stomach. The disorder known as hypochlorhydria (HCL deficiency) can occur in anyone, but becomes increasingly common as we get older. In the event of a clinically significant HCL deficiency, a supplemental form of HCL (known as *betaine hydrochloride*) is sometimes used. This supplement is taken either during or immediately after major meals. It is important to avoid taking excessive quantities of HCL, as this can irritate the stomach. Should you experience any irritation or unusual warmth in the stomach after taking betaine hydrochloride, reduce the dosage until you reach a level where this does not occur.

Please note: Betaine hydrochloride supplements should NOT be taken on an empty stomach and are NOT to be used if you suffer with, or have a history of, stomach or duodenal ulcers without the consent of your doctor.

PANCREATIC ENZYMES

Within the duodenum, pancreatic enzymes are necessary for the digestion of proteins, fats and carbohydrates. The *protease* portion of pancreatic enzymes (such as *chymotrypsin*, *trypsin*, *carboxypeptidase*) digest proteins. Deficiency in these enzymes increases the likelihood of food allergies and encourages the production of toxins such as polyamines. As with HCL, supplemental replacement of pancreatic enzymes (in the form of *pancreatin*) can be a very useful part of the therapy for candidiasis, in that they provide great protection against pathogenic organisms in the small intestine, and many alleviate certain digestive symptoms.

B Vitamins

The nutrient category known as the *B-complex* is comprised of several individual B vitamins. B vitamins often work with others or individually to facilitate metabolic processes (such as energy utilization) and either directly or indirectly play a role in the regulation of body systems (such as the endocrine, nervous, immune and digestive systems).

Research suggests that a deficiency and/or impaired utilization of certain B vitamins (such as B_2, B_6 and folic acid) is not uncommon in candidiasis. This fact, combined with the general benefits of the B-complex, suggests it would be prudent to supplement your diet with additional B vitamins either through a B-complex formulation or a multi-vitamin/mineral supplement. It is important to ensure that any supplement you take which contains B-complex specifies that it is *yeast-free*.

BIOTIN

There is one particular member of the B-complex family where even higher levels of supplementation are considered by many to be appropriate in candidiasis. It is thought that the B vitamin *biotin* may play a role in inhibiting the conversion of the simple yeast form of candida into its mycelial fungal form. However, this observation is based on *in vitro* research, and questions have been raised as to whether oral supplementation provides any significant protection against mycelial conversion.

Antioxidants

The *antioxidant* category of nutrients is of great importance to so many aspects of health. Among other things, antioxidants provide protection and promote the proper functioning of cells and tissues by scavenging and/or neutralizing free radicals and related agents. Such agents can damage and/or inhibit the repair of connective tissue throughout the body, including that which is found in the intestinal walls. This, compounded with the tissue stress caused by intestinal candida overgrowth, would obviously be most counterproductive. Free radicals can also add significantly to the stress on the liver and immune system. In truth, collectively free radicals can harm essentially any cell or tissue in the body, damage any essential compound produced in the body and can interfere with necessary chemical processes. While much focus has rightly been placed on free radical sources found in our environment (such as pollution, ultraviolet rays), a great deal of exposure originates from *within* the body (free radicals are a by-product of normal metabolism).

Many nutrients and plant-derived substances possess powerful free radical scavenging effects. The most well known and some of the most heavily researched include *vitamins A, C* and *E, carotonoids*, and the mineral *selenium*. In addition to antioxidant activity, these nutrients have other nutritional functions, many of which are pertinent to the health and repair of the immune and digestive systems and literally every other system in the body.

In general, antioxidants are vital to the proper activity of the immune system. For instance, vitamin C has displayed an ability to enhance the activity of neutrophils (the major class of white blood cells) in response to candida. In addition to its role in immunity, vitamin C is needed to manufacture collagen, the main protein found in connective tissue.

Vitamin A is necessary for the proper health of the mucous membranes (such as in the intestinal tract) and the immune system, and appears to be deficient in some candidiasis sufferers. Vitamin A can be made from beta carotene in the body, however, some people with candida overgrowth may have difficulty making this conversion effectively. Research has shown that vitamin A deficiency can occur in patients with candida-related problems even when they are not deficient in beta carotene.

Vitamin E plays an important part in the healing of damaged tissue, and works very closely with selenium, which shares many of its functions. Selenium is also a major component (along with glutathione) of the powerful detoxifying enzyme glutathione peroxidase.

The above nutrients can be taken either separately or mixed together as part of an antioxidant combination.

Zinc

The trace mineral *zinc* is one of the most important nutrients of immunity. Zinc is needed for the adequate production and activity of white blood cells, thymus function, thymic hormone activity and so on. It is also necessary for wound healing, general tissue repair and the activity of the stomach acid hydrochloric acid. Certain antioxidant processes in the body require zinc as well. A lack of zinc is known to increase our susceptibility to infection and, not surprisingly, zinc deficiency has been linked with candida-related problems in published research. A vast array of essential chemical reactions in the body require adequate levels of zinc, and as such a deficiency can be especially detrimental to your overall state of health.

Other Nutrients

Aside from those nutrients specifically mentioned above, the intake of minerals such as magnesium and iron and essential fatty acids (*see Chapter 8*) deserve special focus due to either deficiencies or imbalances observed in research.

It is important to take a complete array of all essential

nutrients in ample amounts just to maintain health. The additional challenge candida poses to the body, coupled with the increased tendency for deficiencies in candidiasis sufferers, suggest that special emphasis needs to be directed in this area.

The amounts of essential micronutrients required will typically be in excess (often *far* in excess) of what you could realistically supply even in the best of diets. The restrictive nature of the candida control diet might make this even more the case, additionally so if you have food allergies. As a result, nutritional supplementation is advisable in order to ensure that you are giving your body the best and fastest possible route to recovery (see Table below).

The above-mentioned nutrients, herbs and other natural substances are available as dietary supplements and can generally be found in health food stores and similar outlets specializing in natural health care. The following Table represents a hypothetical programme that outlines the appropriate dietary changes and recommendations for supplements which may be suitable for fighting candidiasis successfully.

Please note: It is important that you consult a qualified health practitioner before beginning this or any other health programme. This information is given merely as an example of the type of programme you might want to consider; it is *not* intended to be prescriptive in nature. Children or pregnant or lactating women should not begin a programme of this (or any) sort without their doctor's supervision.

Avoid or reduce intake of (*see Chapter 8 for the length of time these restrictions may be required*)

- sugar (all forms e.g. sucrose, fructose, glucose, dextrose, maltose, lactose, etc.)
- other natural sweeteners (e.g. honey, molasses, maple/corn/rice syrup, barley malt, etc.)
- alcohol
- vinegar and all pickled foods
- other fermented foods (e.g. soy sauce, sauerkraut, miso, amazake, etc.)
- yeast and yeast-based foods
- malted foods
- mushrooms
- dairy products (except 'live' yoghurt)
- fruit (temporarily)
- dried fruit
- fruit juice
- white flour and white rice
- sorbitol and mannitol
- artificial sweeteners, preservatives, colours and flavours

Possible supplements (adult dosages)

- *lactobacillus acidophilus/bifidobacterium* combination (*L. bulgaricus* optional): 300 million–1 billion organisms *of each* two to three times a day–preferably 30 minutes before meals
- caprylic acid (delayed release): approx. 300 mg, gradually increasing to approx. 1,000 mg with each meal
- goldenseal root: 500–1,500 mg two to three times per day
- pau d'arco: see *page 98* for dosage
- echinacea: 1,000–1,500 mg twice a day
- garlic (preferably as macerate or freeze dried): 500–700 mg two to three times per day
- milk thistle: 70–210 mg of *silymarin* two to three times per day

- psyllium seed husks: 1 g, gradually increasing to 3 g twice a day on an empty stomach, followed by a full glass of water
- digestive enzyme combination: as directed on label
  DO NOT take on an empty stomach. These enzymes should NOT be used by those suffering with ulcers of the digestive system without the consent of their doctor.
- multi-vitamin/mineral (yeast-free containing minimum 40–50 mg B-complex): as directed on label
- multiple mineral combination (amino acid chelated): as directed on label
- antioxidant combination: as directed on label.

REFERENCES

Abe, F. et al., *Mycopathologia* 100 (1987): 37–42

Allun-Jones, V. et al., *Lancet* 2 (1982): 1115–18

Bachur, N. et al., *Cancer Research* 38 (1978): 1,745–50

Beck, C. and Necheles, H., *American Journal of Gastroenterology* 35 (1961): 522–27

Beisel, W. et al., *Journal of the American Medical Association* 245 (1981): 53–58

Bernstein, J. et al., *American Journal of Clinical Nutrition* 30 (1977): 613

Bhandari, N. et al., *British Medical Journal* 298 (1989): 1284–87

Boero, M. et al., *Digestion* 28.3 (1983): 158–63

Canini, F. et al., *Clinical Therapy* 114 (1985): 307–14

Cann, P. et al., *Gut* 25 (1984): 168–73

Chaitow, L., *Candida Albicans – Could Yeast Be Your Problem?* (Thorsons, 1996)

Chin, D. et al., *Journal of Family Practice* 20 (1985): 125–38

Collins, E. and Hardt, P., *Journal of Dairy Science* 63 (1980): 830–32

Colombel, J. et al., *Lancet* 2 (1987): 43

Crook, W., *The Yeast Connection* (Professional Books, 1988)

Dardenne, M. et al., *Proceedings of the National Academy of Science* 79 (1982): 5370–73

Desplaces, A. et al., *Arzneim-Forsch.* 25 (1975): 89

Dowd, P. and Heatley, R., *Clinical Science* 66 (1984): 241–48

Edman, J. et al., *American Journal of Obstetrics and Gynecology* 155.5 (1986): 1082–85

Fantus, B. et al., *Journal of the American Medical Association* 114 (1940): 404–408

Fernandes, C. et al., *Journal of Applied Nutrition* 40.1 (1988): 32–34

Fielding, J. and Kehoe. M., *Irish Journal of Medical Science* 153 (1984): 178–80

Galland, L., *Journal of Orthomolecular Psychiatry* 14 (1985): 50–60

Gay, L., *American Journal of Digestive Disorders* 3 (1937): 326–29

Gershon, H. and Shanks, L., *Canadian Journal of Microbiology* 21 (1975): 1317–21

Gershwin, M. et al., *Journal of the American Geriatric Society* 31 (1983): 374–78

Gorbach, S. et al., *Lancet* 2 (1987): 1519

Grimes, D. *Lancet* 1 (1976): 395–97

Hahn, F. and Ciak, J. *Antibiotics* 3 (1976): 577–88

Higgs, J. and Wells, R., *British Journal of Dermatology* Suppl. 86 (1972): 88–102

Hikino, H. et al., *Planta Medica* 50 (1984): 248–50

Hoffman, D. and Kozak, P., *Journal of Allergy and Clinical Immunology* 63 (1979): 213

Holti, G., in Winner and Hurley (eds.), from *Symposium on Candida Infections* (Livingstone, 1966)

Horowitz, B. et al., *Journal of Reproductive Medicine* 29.7 (1984): 441–43

Infectious Disease News (November 1989): 4

Keeney, E., *Bulletin of Johns Hopkins Hospital* 78 (1946): 333–39

Kroker, G., *Food Allergy and Intolerance* (WB Saunders, 1987)

Kumazawa, Y. et al., *International Journal of Immunopharmacology* 6 (1984): 578–92

Lahiri, S. et al., *Annals of Biochemistry and Experimental Medicine of India* 18 (1958): 95

Leeds, A. *et al.*, *Lancet* 1 (1981): 1075–78

Liu, C. *et al.*, *Chinese Traditional and Herbal Drugs Comm.* 9.36 (1979): 7

Mahajan, V. *et al.*, *Saubouraudia* 20 (1982): 79–81

Manning, A. *et al.*, *Lancet* 2 (1977): 417

Naidovich, L. *et al.*, *Farmatsiya* 24.33 (1976): 5

Narducci, F. *et al.*, *Dig. Dis. Sci.* 30 (1985): 40–44

Neuhauser, I. and Gustus, E., *Archives of Internal Medicine* 93 (1954): 53–60

Niv, M. *et al.*, *Clinical Pediatrics* 2 (1963): 407–11

Poser, G., *Arzneim-Forsch.* 21 (1971): 1209

Preininger, V., in R. H. F. Manske (ed.), *The Alkaloids* Volume XV (Academic Press, 1975)

Ransberger, K., *Arthritis and Rheumatism* 8 (1986): 16–19

Rettger, L. *et al.*, *Lactobacillus Acidophilus: Its Therapeutic Application* (Yale University Press, 1935)

Roesler, J. *et al.*, *International Journal of Immunopharmacology* 13.1 (1991): 27–37

Rubenstein, E. *et al.*, *Gastroenterology* 88 (1985): 927–32

Sabir, M. and Bhide, N., *Indian Journal of Physiology and Pharmacology* 15 (1971): 111–32

Samaranayake, L., *Journal of Oral Pathology* 15 (1986): 61–65

Samaranayake, L. *et al.*, *Journal of Medical Microbiology* 17.1 (1984): 13–22

Sanchez, A. *et al.*, *American Journal of Clinical Nutrition* 26 (1973): 1180–84

Sandhu, D. *et al.*, *Mykosen* 23 (1980): 691–98

Saxena, Q. *et al.*, *Immunology* 52 (1984): 41–48

Schwabe, A. *et al.*, *Journal of Applied Physiology* 19 (1964): 335–37

Shahani, K. and Friend, B., *Journal of Applied Nutrition* 36 (1984): 125–52

Stimpel, M., *et al.*, *Infection Immunity* 46 (1984): 845–49

Subbaiah, T. and Amin, A., *Nature* 215 (1967): 527

Truss, C. O., *The Missing Diagnosis* (1983; available from the author: P.O. Box 26508, Birmingham, Alabama 35226, USA)

—, *Journal of Orthomolecular Psychiatry* 13 (1984): 66–93

Vahouny, G. and Kritchevsky, D., *Dietary Fibre in Health and Disease* (New York: Plenum Press, 1982)

Vogel, G. *et al.*, *Toxicology and Applied Pharmacology* 51 (1984): 265

Wacker, A. and Hilbig, W., *Planta Medica* 33 (1978): 89–102

Wagner, V. *et al.*, *Arzneim-Forsch.* 35 (1985): 1069–75

Wagner, V. and Proksch, A., *Economic Medicinal Plant Research* 1 (1985): 113–53

Will, T., *Lancet* 2 (1979): 482

Worthington, B. *et al.*, *Dig. Dis. Sci.* 23 (1978): 23–32

Yamaguchi, H., *Saubouraudia* 12.3 (1974): 320–28

Of further interest…

Recipes for Health: Candida Albicans

FEATURING OVER 100 SUGAR-FREE AND YEAST-FREE RECIPES

SHIRLEY TRICKETT

Thrush, sinusitis, allergies, throat infections, depression, bloating, food cravings, weight problems, chronic muscle pain – these are just some of the conditions associated with an overproduction of the yeast candida albicans in the body.

This practical self-help guide explains:

what causes candida growth and how to prevent it
which foods to eat and which foods to avoid

Shirley Trickett includes over 100 easy-to-prepare recipes which are low in refined carbohydrates, virtually yeast-free and full of flavour, and features everyday ingredients which are readily available and economical to use.

It is a cookbook guaranteed to improve your health and well-being.

Candida Albicans

LEON CHAITOW

Candida albicans is a yeast which exists inside all of us and normally presents no problems, but today's widespread use of broad spectrum antibiotics, contraceptive pills and steroids, as well as a sugar-rich diet, can cause a proliferation of this parasite yeast.

Its spread can often be the root cause of a wide variety of problems – ME/chronic fatigue syndrome; depression; anxiety; irritability; diarrhoea; bloatedness; heartburn; tiredness; allergies; acne; migraine; cystitis; menstrual problems, etc. Leon Chaitow shows how to detect whether yeast is your problem, and provides a comprehensive and non-drug programme for its control.

Leon Chaitow, osteopath, naturopath and acupuncturist, is a leading international practitioner and successful author of a wide range of health books.

RECIPES FOR HEALTH:
CANDIDA ALBICANS   0 7225 2967 8   £5.99   ☐
CANDIDA ALBICANS   0 7225 3343 8   £3.99   ☐

All these books are available from your local bookseller or can be ordered direct from the publishers.

To order direct just tick the titles you want and fill in the form below:

Name: _____

Address: _____

_____

_____ Postcode: _____

Send to Thorsons Mail Order, Dept 3, HarperCollins*Publishers*, Westerhill Road, Bishopbriggs, Glasgow G64 2QT.

Please enclose a cheque or postal order or your authority to debit your Visa/Access account –

Credit card no: _____

Expiry date: _____

Signature: _____

– up to the value of the cover price plus:

UK & BFPO: Add £1.00 for the first book and 25p for each additional book ordered.

Overseas orders including Eire: Please add £2.95 service charge. Books will be sent by surface mail but quotes for airmail dispatches will be given on request.

24-HOUR TELEPHONE ORDERING SERVICE FOR ACCESS/VISA CARDHOLDERS – TEL: 0141 772 2281.